Disorders of Puberty

Disorders of Puberty

The Causes and the Endocrine Medical Treatment

Special Issue Editors

Sandro La Vignera
Aldo E. Calogero

MDPI • Basel • Beijing • Wuhan • Barcelona • Belgrade • Manchester • Tokyo • Cluj • Tianjin

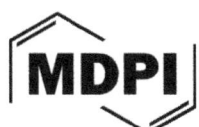

Special Issue Editors
Sandro La Vignera
University of Catania
Italy

Aldo E. Calogero
University of Catania
Italy

Editorial Office
MDPI
St. Alban-Anlage 66
4052 Basel, Switzerland

This is a reprint of articles from the Special Issue published online in the open access journal *Journal of Clinical Medicine* (ISSN 2077-0383) (available at: https://www.mdpi.com/journal/jcm/special_issues/Disorders_Puberty).

For citation purposes, cite each article independently as indicated on the article page online and as indicated below:

LastName, A.A.; LastName, B.B.; LastName, C.C. Article Title. *Journal Name* **Year**, *Article Number*, Page Range.

ISBN 978-3-03936-196-0 (Pbk)
ISBN 978-3-03936-197-7 (PDF)

© 2020 by the authors. Articles in this book are Open Access and distributed under the Creative Commons Attribution (CC BY) license, which allows users to download, copy and build upon published articles, as long as the author and publisher are properly credited, which ensures maximum dissemination and a wider impact of our publications.

The book as a whole is distributed by MDPI under the terms and conditions of the Creative Commons license CC BY-NC-ND.

Contents

About the Special Issue Editors vii

Preface to "Disorders of Puberty" ix

Sandro La Vignera, Rossella Cannarella, Rosita A. Condorelli and Aldo E. Calogero
Disorders of Puberty: Endocrinology of the Pre-Pubertal Testis
Reprinted from: *J. Clin. Med.* 2020, 9, 780, doi:10.3390/jcm9030780 1

Rossella Cannarella, Iva Arato, Rosita A. Condorelli, Giovanni Luca, Federica Barbagallo, Angela Alamo, Catia Bellucci, Cinzia Lilli, Sandro La Vignera, Riccardo Calafiore, Francesca Mancuso and Aldo E. Calogero
The IGF1 Receptor Is Involved in Follicle-Stimulating Hormone Signaling in Porcine Neonatal Sertoli Cells
Reprinted from: *J. Clin. Med.* 2019, 8, 577, doi:10.3390/jcm8050577 5

Rossella Cannarella, Francesca Mancuso, Rosita A. Condorelli, Iva Arato, Laura M. Mongioì, Filippo Giacone, Cinzia Lilli, Catia Bellucci, Sandro La Vignera, Riccardo Calafiore, Giovanni Luca and Aldo E. Calogero
Effects of GH and IGF1 on Basal and FSH-Modulated Porcine Sertoli Cells In-Vitro
Reprinted from: *J. Clin. Med.* 2019, 8, 811, doi:10.3390/jcm8060811 15

Rossella Cannarella, Iva Arato, Rosita A. Condorelli, Laura M. Mongioì, Cinzia Lilli, Catia Bellucci, Sandro La Vignera, Giovanni Luca, Francesca Mancuso and Aldo E. Calogero
Effects of Insulin on Porcine Neonatal Sertoli Cell Responsiveness to FSH In Vitro
Reprinted from: *J. Clin. Med.* 2019, 8, 809, doi:10.3390/jcm8060809 25

Anna Perri, Danilo Lofaro, Giulia Izzo, Benedetta Aquino, Massimo Bitonti, Giuseppe Ciambrone, Sandro La Vignera, Carlotta Pozza, Daniele Gianfrilli and Antonio Aversa
The Risky Health Behaviours of Male Adolescents in the Southern Italian Region: Implications for Sexual and Reproductive Disease
Reprinted from: *J. Clin. Med.* 2019, 8, 1414, doi:10.3390/jcm8091414 37

Ylenia Duca, Antonio Aversa, Rosita Angela Condorelli, Aldo Eugenio Calogero and Sandro La Vignera
Substance Abuse and Male Hypogonadism
Reprinted from: *J. Clin. Med.* 2019, 8, 732, doi:10.3390/jcm8050732 47

Ylenia Duca, Andrea Di Cataldo, Giovanna Russo, Emanuela Cannata, Giovanni Burgio, Michele Compagnone, Angela Alamo, Rosita A. Condorelli, Sandro La Vignera and Aldo E. Calogero
Testicular Function of Childhood Cancer Survivors: Who Is Worse?
Reprinted from: *J. Clin. Med.* 2019, 8, 2204, doi:10.3390/jcm8122204 73

Rosita A. Condorelli, Sandro La Vignera, Laura M. Mongioì, Angela Alamo, Filippo Giacone, Rossella Cannarella and Aldo E. Calogero
Thyroid Hormones and Spermatozoa: In Vitro Effects on Sperm Mitochondria, Viability and DNA Integrity
Reprinted from: *J. Clin. Med.* 2019, 8, 756, doi:10.3390/jcm8050756 85

Rosita A. Condorelli, Aldo E. Calogero, Rossella Cannarella, Filippo Giacone, Laura M. Mongioi', Laura Cimino, Antonio Aversa and Sandro La Vignera
Poor Efficacy of L-Acetylcarnitine in the Treatment of Asthenozoospermia in Patients with Type 1 Diabetes
Reprinted from: *J. Clin. Med.* **2019**, *8*, 585, doi:10.3390/jcm8050585 . . . . **93**

Rossella Cannarella, Aldo E. Calogero, Rosita A. Condorelli, Filippo Giacone, Antonio Aversa and Sandro La Vignera
Management and Treatment of Varicocele in Children and Adolescents: An Endocrinologic Perspective
Reprinted from: *J. Clin. Med.* **2019**, *8*, 1410, doi:10.3390/jcm8091410 . . . . **101**

Sandro La Vignera, Rosita A. Condorelli, Laura Cimino, Rossella Cannarella, Filippo Giacone and Aldo E. Calogero
Early Identification of Isolated Sertoli Cell Dysfunction in Prepubertal and Transition Age: Is It Time?
Reprinted from: *J. Clin. Med.* **2019**, *8*, 636, doi:10.3390/jcm8050636 . . . . **113**

About the Special Issue Editors

Sandro La Vignera. Born in Catania, Italy, on the 27th of July 1977. He earned his M.D. in 2002 at the University of Catania reporting 110/110 with honors, his post-graduate degree in Endocrinology in 2007 reporting 70/70 with honors, and Ph.D. in Andrological Science, Human Reproduction, and Biotechnologies in 2012. Since 2014, he has been Assistant Professor and Physician of Endocrinology at the University Teaching Hospital "Policlinico-Vittorio Emanuele", University of Catania. He has also been awarded the National Scientific Qualification as Full Professor of Endocrinology. Orcid number: 0000-0002-7113-2372. He has authored over 240 publications in peer-reviewed journals on Pubmed. h-Index: 28 (Scopus). His research activity has mainly focused on the endocrinological aspects of reproduction and human sexuality, including male accessory gland infections/inflammations, hypogonadism, benign prostatic hyperplasia, and the impact of thyroid dysfunction on semen quality. He has been awarded as Best Under 40 Researcher in 2017 by the Italian Society of Endocrinology and included in the "Top Worldwide Scientists Database" in 2019 by Plos Biology. He holds important positions with several scientific societies and journals. He is a Board Member of the Master of Reproductive Biotechnology of the University of Catania, Delegate for the Sicilian Regional Health Department for continuing medical education, Treasurer of the Italian Society of Andrology and Medicine of Sexuality, Member of the Regional Executive Council of the Italian Society of Endocrinology, Member of the Editorial Board of *Scientific Reports-Nature* and *Annals of Translational Medicine* and *Androgens: Clinical Research and Therapeutics*, and Guest Editor for the *Journal of Clinical Medicine* and *Frontiers in Endocrinology*.

Aldo E. Calogero. Born in Vittoria (RG), Italy, on the 29th of December 1958, Prof. Calogero earned his M.D. degree in 1983 at the University of Catania, reporting 110/110 with honors. In 1986, he achieved a post-graduate degree in Endocrinology at the University of Catania reporting 50/50 with honors. Orcid number: 0000-0001-6950-335X. Currently, he is Full Professor of Endocrinology and Metabolic Diseases and Director of the Division of Endocrinology, University Teaching Hospital "Policlinico-Vittorio Emanuele", University of Catania, Italy. He has published more than 800 articles, book chapters, and abstracts; of which, 385 are original articles published in peer-reviewed journals with impact factor (total impact factor 1277.474, 2018). h-Index: 52 (Scopus). He has organized and participated in the organization of numerous national and international conferences and has been a speaker and chairperson at more than 250 national and international congresses. He was included in the "Top Worldwide Scientists Database" in 2019 by Plos Biology. Prof. Calogero's research activity was initially dedicated to the neuroendocrinological aspects of CRH- and GnRH-secreting neurons, which were investigated using in-vitro and in-vivo experimental models at the National Institute of Health (Bethesda, MD, USA). Subsequently, it was extended to different areas of male infertility that included sperm chromosome and DNA integrity, cigarette smoke, male accessory gland infections/inflammations (MAGI), diabetes and metabolic disorders, hypogonadism, and hormonal and non-hormonal treatment of male infertility. In particular, a great number of studies have been carried out to demonstrate the negative impact of MAGI, pollutants, diabetes, and cigarette smoke on sperm parameters, leading to the development of preventive strategies. Recently, he has also been studying the possible existence of a male equivalent of polycystic ovary syndrome.

Preface to "Disorders of Puberty"

This book was conceived to help understand the mechanisms that occur in childhood and whose alterations probably contribute to the pathogenesis of male idiopathic infertility, a very common condition in our society. We hope that the topics contribute to the correct management of andrological health from the first months of life and then in childhood and adolescence, to correct harmful lifestyles, and to develop diagnostic and therapeutic strategies suitable for achieving an important goal, to protect the health of the fathers of tomorrow! Among these, a close collaboration between pediatricians, endocrinologists, and andrologists must certainly be considered. Finally, we are deeply indebted to Prof. Rosita A. Condorelli and Dr. Rossella Cannarella for their valuable and enthusiastic contribution without which this book would not have been possible.

Sandro La Vignera, Aldo E. Calogero
Special Issue Editors

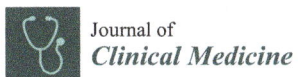 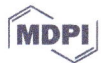

Editorial

Disorders of Puberty: Endocrinology of the Pre-Pubertal Testis

Sandro La Vignera, Rossella Cannarella, Rosita A. Condorelli and Aldo E. Calogero *

Department of Clinical and Experimental Medicine, University of Catania, 95123 Catania, Italy; sandrolavignera@unict.it (S.L.V.); rossella.cannarella@phd.unict.it (R.C.); rosita.condorelli@unict.it (R.A.C.)
* Correspondence: acaloger@unict.it; Tel.: +39-95-378-2641

Received: 11 March 2020; Accepted: 11 March 2020; Published: 13 March 2020

Abstract: Male infertility is a widespread condition among western countries. Meta-regression data show that sperm concentration and total sperm count have halved in the last decades. The reasons of this decline are still unclear. The evaluation of testicular function in pre-pubertal children may be effective in the timely detection of Sertoli cell (SC) dysfunction, which anticipates the diagnosis of male infertility. The aim of this Special Issue is to gather together in vitro evidence on SC physiology, causes of SC dysfunction, and to suggest a practical approach to be adopted in children.

Keywords: Sertoli cells; Sertoli cell dysfunction; male infertility; inhibin B; AMH; IGF1; insulin

---

The endocrinology of pre-pubertal testis represents a challenge for both endocrinologists and pediatricians because the testis has been believed to be dormant before the activation of the hypothalamic-pituitary-gonadal axis. However, various metabolic processes occur in the testis before the onset of puberty; these include proliferation of Sertoli cells (SC), secretion of anti-Müllerian hormone (AMH), and a slight increase in testicular volume. In particular, it is debated whether any of these parameters may be used as a useful diagnostic marker to identify early SC dysfunction, which probably anticipates the diagnosis of infertility in adulthood. This Special Issue focuses on the most recent advances in the endocrinology of the testis in pre-pubertal and transitional ages. The aim is to evaluate the physiology of pre-pubertal SCs and provide a proposal for the early detection of SC dysfunction. The structure of the Special Issue includes three reviews and seven original articles (including clinical and preclinical studies).

Pre-clinical studies mainly deal with the role of the growth hormone (GH)-insulin-like growth factor 1 (IGF1) axis on SCs. For these kinds of studies, SCs from pre-pubertal pigs were cultured. In contrast to adult SCs, pre-pubertal ones are immature, are able to proliferate, and can secret AMH and inhibin B hormones in the incubation medium. In the adult stage, SCs are mature, have lost the ability to proliferate, and therefore, these cells cannot be cultured. Pre-pubertal porcine SCs represent the in vitro system most similar to children's SCs. Cannarella et al. report, for the first time, the role of the IGF1 receptor (IGF1R) in SCs, where they play a role similar to that already found in granulosa cells [1]. Other in vitro studies in this Special Issue [2,3] evaluate how incubation with follicle-stimulating hormone (FSH), GH, IGF1, or insulin impacts SC proliferation, AMH, and inhibin B secretion. Interestingly, these findings somehow question the role of FSH in SC proliferation in vitro, since no proliferative effect was found after 48 h of incubation. In contrast, both IGF1 and insulin enhanced SC proliferation. These results suggest that highly complex molecular mechanisms are involved in SC proliferation, and AMH and inhibin secretion in vivo. More than the effect of FSH alone, the increase in testicular volume and amount of circulating AMH and inhibin B in pre-pubertal children likely reflect a combination of multiple hormonal stimuli, among which IGF1 may play a relevant role.

As far the clinical aspects, childhood cancer [4], pediatric varicocele [5], and risky lifestyles [6] (including substance abuse [7]) are addressed in the current Special Issue. Duca et al. [...] evaluate the testicular function of childhood cancer survivors and address which cancer, therapy, and age of treatment has the worst reproductive outcomes in adulthood. This topic is of particular interest since the drugs used in pediatric oncology are very effective in terms of survival. Because childhood cancer survivors often will seek fertility later in life, it is wiser to use drugs with the lowest toxicity for the reproductive apparatus. The management of pediatric varicocele is somehow a debated issue. In the review by Cannarella et al., a general overview of pediatric varicocele is given, including a compelling flowchart reporting the management from an endocrinologic point of view [5]. Interestingly, a survey of the risky lifestyles for the reproductive and sexual function in male adolescents is provided by Perri et al. [6]. Worryingly, this study reveals a non-negligible percentage of smokers, drinkers, and cannabis consumers among male adolescents. In addition, many of them ignore sexual transmitted infections; proper information about risky health behaviors should be given.

Therapeutic issues are also addressed in this Special Issue. These include the effectiveness of L-acetyl-carnitine for the treatment of asthenozoospermia in patients with type I diabetes mellitus [8] and the in vitro effects of thyroid hormones in sperm mitochondrial function, viability, and DNA integrity [9].

Finally, La Vignera et al. [10] discuss the diagnostic management that may be adopted to identify the early signs of isolated SC dysfunction. Therapeutic possibilities are also discussed. Overall, this study highlights the importance of carrying out well-designed prospective studies to validate the proposal made in the every-day clinical practice. Briefly, we suggest assessing pre-pubertal markers of testicular function (AMH and inhibin B) and testicular volume in patients with risk factors such as those detailed in Figure 1. Sperm analysis should not be requested earlier than 1.5 years of puberty onset [10]. As suggested in this article, measuring the response of AMH to stimulation with FSH, despite deserving a clinical validation, can represent a diagnostic test to promptly identify Sertolian dysfunction in the pre-pubertal age.

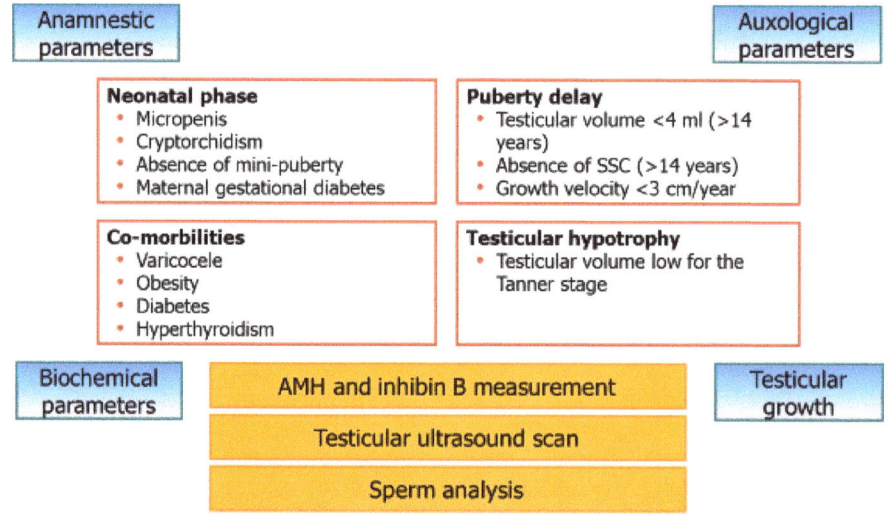

Figure 1. Diagnostic flow-chart for the early detection of Sertoli cell dysfunction. Children or transitional age adolescents showing anamnestic or physical signs at risk for Sertoli cell (SC) dysfunction should undergo to the assessment of biochemical parameters, testicular ultrasound and, whenever possible, sperm analysis.

Author Contributions: Conceptualization, S.L.V.; project administration, A.E.C.; supervision, R.A.C.; writing—original draft: R.C., writing—review & editing, S.L.V. and A.E.C. All authors have read and agreed to the published version of the manuscript.

Funding: This research received no external funding.

Conflicts of Interest: The authors declare no conflict of interest.

References

1. Cannarella, R.; Arato, I.; Condorelli, R.A.; Luca, G.; Barbagallo, F.; Alamo, A.; Bellucci, C.; Lilli, C.; La Vignera, S.; Calafiore, R.; et al. The IGF1 Receptor Is Involved in Follicle-Stimulating Hormone Signaling in Porcine Neonatal Sertoli Cells. *J. Clin. Med.* **2019**, *8*, 577. [CrossRef] [PubMed]
2. Cannarella, R.; Mancuso, F.; Condorelli, R.A.; Arato, I.; Mongioì, L.M.; Giacone, F.; Lilli, C.; Bellucci, C.; La Vignera, S.; Calafiore, R.; et al. Effects of GH and IGF1 on Basal and FSH-Modulated Porcine Sertoli Cells In Vitro. *J. Clin. Med.* **2019**, *8*, 811. [CrossRef] [PubMed]
3. Cannarella, R.; Arato, I.; Condorelli, R.A.; Mongioì, L.M.; Lilli, C.; Bellucci, C.; La Vignera, S.; Luca, G.; Mancuso, F.; Calogero, A.E. Effects of Insulin on Porcine Neonatal Sertoli Cell Responsiveness to FSH In Vitro. *J. Clin. Med.* **2019**, *8*, 809. [CrossRef] [PubMed]
4. Duca, Y.; Di Cataldo, A.; Russo, G.; Cannata, E.; Burgio, G.; Compagnone, M.; Alamo, A.; Condorelli, R.A.; La Vignera, S.; Calogero, A.E. Testicular Function of Childhood Cancer Survivors: Who Is Worse? *J. Clin. Med.* **2019**, *8*, 2204. [CrossRef] [PubMed]
5. Cannarella, R.; Calogero, A.E.; Condorelli, R.A.; Giacone, F.; Aversa, A.; La Vignera, S. Management and Treatment of Varicocele in Children and Adolescents: An Endocrinologic Perspective. *J. Clin. Med.* **2019**, *8*, 1410. [CrossRef] [PubMed]
6. Perri, A.; Lofaro, D.; Izzo, G.; Aquino, B.; Bitonti, M.; Ciambrone, G.; La Vignera, S.; Pozza, C.; Gianfrilli, D.; Aversa, A. The Risky Health Behaviours of Male Adolescents in the Southern Italian Region: Implications for Sexual and Reproductive Disease. *J. Clin. Med.* **2019**, *8*, 1414. [CrossRef] [PubMed]
7. Duca, Y.; Aversa, A.; Condorelli, R.A.; Calogero, A.E.; La Vignera, S. Substance Abuse and Male Hypogonadism. *J. Clin. Med.* **2019**, *8*, 732. [CrossRef] [PubMed]
8. Condorelli, R.A.; Calogero, A.E.; Cannarella, R.; Giacone, F.; Mongioi', L.M.; Cimino, L.; Aversa, A.; La Vignera, S. Poor Efficacy of L-Acetylcarnitine in the Treatment of Asthenozoospermia in Patients with Type 1 Diabetes. *J. Clin. Med.* **2019**, *8*, 585. [CrossRef] [PubMed]
9. Condorelli, R.A.; La Vignera, S.; Mongioì, L.M.; Alamo, A.; Giacone, F.; Cannarella, R.; Calogero, A.E. Thyroid Hormones and Spermatozoa: In VitroEffects on Sperm Mitochondria, Viability and DNA Integrity. *J. Clin. Med.* **2019**, *8*, 756. [CrossRef] [PubMed]
10. La Vignera, S.; Condorelli, R.A.; Cimino, L.; Cannarella, R.; Giacone, F.; Calogero, A.E. Early Identification of Isolated Sertoli Cell Dysfunction in Prepubertal and Transition Age: Is It Time? *J. Clin. Med.* **2019**, *8*, 636. [CrossRef] [PubMed]

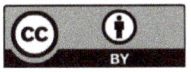

© 2020 by the authors. Licensee MDPI, Basel, Switzerland. This article is an open access article distributed under the terms and conditions of the Creative Commons Attribution (CC BY) license (http://creativecommons.org/licenses/by/4.0/).

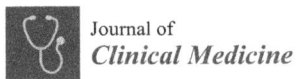

Article

The IGF1 Receptor Is Involved in Follicle-Stimulating Hormone Signaling in Porcine Neonatal Sertoli Cells

Rossella Cannarella [1,*,†], Iva Arato [2,†], Rosita A. Condorelli [1], Giovanni Luca [2], Federica Barbagallo [1], Angela Alamo [1], Catia Bellucci [2], Cinzia Lilli [2], Sandro La Vignera [1], Riccardo Calafiore [3], Francesca Mancuso [2,‡] and Aldo E. Calogero [1,‡]

1   Department of Clinical and Experimental Medicine, University of Catania, 95123 Catania, Italy; rosita.condorelli@unict.it (R.A.C.); federica.barbagallo11@gmail.com (F.B.); angela.alamo1986@gmail.com (A.A.); sandrolavignera@unict.it (S.L.V.); acaloger@unict.it (A.E.C.)
2   Department of Experimental Medicine, University of Perugia, 06123 Perugia, Italy; iva.arato@libero.it (I.A.); giovanni.luca@unipg.it (G.L.); catia.bellucci@unipg.it (C.B.); cinzia.lilli@unipg.it (C.L.); francesca.mancuso@unipg.it (F.M.)
3   Department of Medicine, University of Perugia, 06123 Perugia, Italy; riccardo.calafiore@unipg.it
*   Correspondence: roxcannarella@gmail.com; Tel.: +39-389-5986660
†   These authors contributed equally to this article.
‡   These authors share the senior authorship of this article.

Received: 21 March 2019; Accepted: 24 April 2019; Published: 27 April 2019

Abstract: Experimental evidence has shown that the IGF1 receptor (IGF1R) is involved in testicular development during embryogenesis. More recently, data gathered from mice granulosa cells and zebrafish spermatogonia suggest that IGF1R has a role in Follicle-stimulating hormone (FSH) signaling. No evidence has been reported on this matter in Sertoli cells (SCs) so far. The aim of the study was to evaluate the role, if any, of the IGF1R in FSH signaling in SCs. The effects of FSH exposure on myosin-phosphatase 1 (MYPT1), ERK 1/2, AKT^{308}, AKT^{473}, c-Jun N-terminal kinase (JNK) phosphorylation and on anti-Müllerian hormone (AMH), inhibin B and FSH receptor (FSHR) mRNA levels were assessed with and without the IGF1R inhibitor NVP-AEW541 in purified and functional porcine neonatal SCs. Pre-treatment with NVP-AEW541 inhibited the FSH-induced MYPT1 and ERK 1/2 phosphorylation, decreased the FSH-dependent Protein kinase B $(AKT)^{308}$ phosphorylation, but did not affect the FSH-induced AKT^{473} and JNK phosphorylation rate. It also interfered with the FSH-induced AMH and FSHR down-regulation. No influence was observed on the FSH-stimulated Inhibin B gene expression. Conclusion. These findings support the role of theIGF1R in FSH signaling in porcine SCs. The possible influence of IGF1 stimulation on the FSH-mediated effects on SCs should be further explored.

Keywords: Follicle-stimulating hormone; Insulin-like growth factor 1; Insulin-like growth factor 1 receptor; Sertoli cells; infertility

---

1. Introduction

Follicle-stimulating hormone (FSH) is required for normal spermatogenesis [1]. A deeper insight into the molecular mechanisms involved in FSH signaling in Sertoli cells (SCs) might help to elucidate some cases of unexplained male infertility. As for many G protein-coupled receptors (GPCRs), the FSH receptor (FSHR), once over stimulated by FSH, triggers Gαs, which activates the adenylate cyclase, resulting in increased intracellular cAMP levels. The latter leads to protein kinase A (PKA) activation, which in turn stimulates many different transcription factors [2].

A number of studies have assigned a role in SC function to the insulin-like growth factor 1 receptor (IGF1R), which belongs to the tyrosine kinases receptor family [3]. Accordingly, the IGF1R is expressed in SCs and is required for testis development [4] and SC proliferation [5].

The phosphatidylinositol-3 kinase (PI3K) signaling, involving AKT phosphorylation, is required for cell transcription, translation, proliferation and apoptosis [6]. PI3K, which is classically activated by tyrosine kinases receptors such as IGF1R [7], is also stimulated by several GPCRs. The mechanisms through which GPCRs are able to activate PI3K are less understood compared with the classical activation by tyrosine kinases receptors [6]. The PI3K/AKT pathway has been showed to be required for the FSH-dependent gene expression regulation [8]. Recently, FSH has been shown to activate the PI3K in a PKA-dependent manner [9]. Some evidence suggests that the mechanism through which FSH activate the PI3K/AKT signaling may entail the IGF1R. Accordingly, a study carried out in mouse granulosa cells showed a lack of FSH-induced AKT phosphorylation in NVP-AEW541 (an IGF1R inhibitor) pre-treated cells, thus suggesting that the IGF1R is required for FSH signaling [8]. Similar findings have been reported in spermatogonia from zebrafish [10].

The protein phosphatase 1β (PP1β) has been regarded as the possible hub linking between the FSH and the IGF1R signaling in granulosa cells [8]. PP1 is an ubiquitous eukaryotic Ser/Thr phosphatase involved in the regulation of various cell functions. The substrate specificity is given by the binding of the regulatory subunit to the PP1 catalytic subunit (PP1c). The myosin-phosphatase 1 (MYPT1) is a protein made up by three subunits: the PP1c, a targeting/regulatory subunit and a 20kDa subunit of unknown function called M20 [11,12]. PP1 and MYPT1 have been found to be associated with IRS1 in mouse granulosa cells [13]. Furthermore, PKA is known to activate PP1 through MYPT1 phosphorylation [13]. Incubation with tautomycim, a selective PP1β inhibitor, has been shown to inhibit FSH-mediated IRS1 phosphorylation, in the presence of endogenous IGF1 in granulosa cells [8].

The role of the IGF1R in FSH signaling has not been investigated in SCs so far. Therefore, this study was undertaken to explore this topic. To accomplish this, we evaluated the effects of FSH on MYPT1^{668}, ERK 1/2, AKT^{308}, AKT^{473}, JNK phosphorylation in purified and functional porcine neonatal SCs, with and without pre-treatment with the IGF1R inhibitor NVP-AEW541 and the PP1β inhibitor tautomycin. We also investigated whether the FSH-dependent AMH, Inhibin B and FSHR gene expression was influenced by pre-treatment with the IGF1R inhibitor NVP-AEW541.

2. Experimental Section

2.1. Ethics Statement

This study was conducted in strict compliance with the Guide for the Care and Use of Laboratory Animals of the National Institutes of Health and Perugia University Animal Care. The protocol was approved by the internal Institutional Ethic Committee (Ministry of Health authorization n. 971/2015-PR, 9/14/2015).

2.2. Sertoli Cell Isolation, Culture, Characterization and Function

SCs were obtained from neonatal prepubertal Large White pigs at 7–15 days of age. From each testis, we isolated 60×10^6 SCs with a 95% of purity and a negligible percentage of contaminant cells (Leydig and Peritubular cells < 5%), using established methods [14,15]. Briefly, after removing the fibrous capsule, the testes were finely chopped and digested twice enzymatically, with a mixed solution of trypsin and deoxyribonuclease I (DNase I) in Hank's Balanced Salt Solution (HBSS; Merck KGaA, Darmstadt, Germany) and collagenase P (Roche Diagnostics S.p.A., Monza, Italy). The tissue pellet was centrifuged passed through a 500-μm pore stainless steel mesh, and then resuspended in glycine to eliminate residual Leydig and peritubular cells [16]. The resulting pellet was collected and maintained in HAM's F12 medium (Euroclone, Milan, Italy), supplemented with 0.166 nmol l−1 retinoic acid, (Sigma-Aldrich, Darmstadt, Germany) and 5 mL per 500 mL insulin-transferrin-selenium (ITS, Becton Dickinson cat. no. 354352; Franklin Lakes, NJ, USA) in 95% air/5% CO_2 at 37 °C. After three days in culture, the purity and the functional competence of SC monolayers were performed according to previously established methods [17].

2.3. Culture and Treatment

When the SC monolayers were confluent (at three days of culture), they underwent the following treatments: (1) dimethyl sulfoxide (DMSO) or NVP-AE541 for 1 h and then incubated with vehicle or urofollitropin (hpFSH) (Fostimon®, IBSA Farmaceutici Srl, Rome, Italy) at the concentration of 50 ng/mL for 15 min; (2) DMSO or 1 µM tautomycin for 5.5 h, followed by vehicle or hpFSH (50 ng/mL) for 15 min; (3) DMSO or 1 µM tautomycin for 5.5 h and NVP-AEW541 for 1 h, followed by vehicle or hpFSH (50 ng/mL) for 15 min, as described elsewhere [16]. Cultures were maintained in humidified atmosphere of 95% air/5% CO_2 at 34 °C.

2.4. Western Blot Analysis

At the end of the incubation period, total cell lysates were collected in radioimmunoprecipitation assay (RIPA) lysis buffer (Santa Cruz Biotechnology Inc., Santa Cruz, CA, USA). The mixture was centrifuged at 1000× *g* (Eppendorf, NY, USA) for 10 min, the supernatant was collected and total protein content was measured by the Bradford method [18]. Sample aliquots were stored at −20 °C for Western blot (WB) analysis. The cell extracts were separated by 4%–12% SDS-PAGE and equal amounts of protein (70 µg protein/lane) were run and blotted on nitrocellulose membranes (BioRad, Hercules, CA, USA). The membranes were incubated overnight in a buffer containing 10 mM Tris(Hydroxymethyl)aminomethane (TRIS), 0.5 M NaCl, 1% (v/v) Tween 20 (Sigma-Aldrich), rabbit 3048 anti-pospho-MYPT1 (Ser 668) (dilution factor 1:1000) (Cell Signaling), rabbit PA5-17164 anti-myosin-phosphatase 1 (MYPT1) (dilution factor 1:1000) (ThermoFisher), rabbit 13038 anti-phospho-AKT (Thr308) (dilution factor 1:1000) (Cell Signaling), rabbit 9271 anti-phospho-AKT (Ser473) (dilution factor 1:1000) (Cell Signaling), rabbit 9272 anti-AKT (dilution factor 1:1000) (Cell Signaling), mouse 05-481 anti-phospho-ERK Kinase1/2 (dilution factor 1:100) (Millipore Merck), ABS44 rabbit anti-ERK 1/2 (dilution factor 1:2000) (Millipore Merck), rabbit 07-175 anti-phospho-JNK (Thr18/Tyr185,Thr221/Tyr223) (dilution factor 1:500) (Millipore Merck), rabbit 06-748 anti-JNK (dilution factor 1:1000) (Millipore Merck), mouse anti-Glyceraldehyde-3-Phosphate Dehydrogenase (GADPH) (6C5): sc-32233 (dilution factor 1:200) (Santa Cruz) primary antibodies. Primary antibody binding was then detected by incubating the membranes for an additional 60 min in a buffer containing horseradish peroxidase conjugated anti-rabbit (Sigma-Aldrich; dilution factor, 1:5000) and/or anti-mouse (Santa Cruz Biotechnology Inc.; dilution factor, 1:5000) IgG secondary antibodies. The bands were detected by enhanced chemiluminescence.

2.5. Reverse Transcription Polymerase Chain Reaction Analysis

Total RNA was extracted and quantified by reading the optical density at 260 nm. In particular, 2.5 µg of total RNA was subjected to reverse transcription (RT, Thermo Scientific, Waltham, MA, USA) to a final volume of 20 µL. The qPCR was performed using 50 ng of the cDNA prepared by RT and a SYBR Green Master Mix (Stratagene, Amsterdam, The Netherlands–Agilent Technology). This was performed in an Mx3000P cycler (Stratagene), using FAM for detection and ROX as the reference dye.

The following primers were used for real-time PCR analysis: AMH, forward primers 5′-GCGAACTTAGCGTGGACCTG-3′, revers primers 5′-CTTGGCAGTTGTTGGCTTGATATG-3′; Inhibin B, forward primers 5′-TGGCTGGAGTGACTGGAT-3′, revers primers 5′-CCGTGTGGAAGGATGAGG-3′; FSHR forward primers 5′-TTTCACAGTCGCCCTCTTTCCC-3′, revers primers 5′-TGAGTATAGCAGCCACAGATGACC-3′; actin, forward primers 5′-ATGGTGGGTATGGGTCAGAA-3′, revers primers 5′-CTTCTCCATGTCGTCCCAGT-3′.

2.6. Statistical Analysis

Results are shown as mean ± SD throughout the study. Data were analyzed for statistical significance by one-way ANOVA, followed by Tukey post hoc test using SPSS 9.0 for Windows (SPSS Inc., Chicago, IL, USA). A statistically significant difference was accepted when the p value was lower than 0.05.

3. Results

To elucidate whether the IGF1R and PP1β are involved in FSH signaling, we investigated if the FSH-dependent MYPT1, AKT and JNK phosphorylation was affected by pre-treatment with NPV-AEW541 (an IGF1R inhibitor) and/or tautomycin (a PP1β inhibitor). To further analyze the role of the IGF1R on the FSH-dependent AMH and inhibin B gene expression, we evaluated AMH and inhibin B mRNA levels in the FSH-incubated plates, with and without pre-treatment with NPV-AEW541.

3.1. Western Blot Analysis

Treatment with FSH increased the MYPT1668/MYPT1 phosphorylation ratio. This effect was inhibited by pre-treatment with NVP-AEW541 and/or tautomycin (Figure 1, panels a and b). FSH increased ERK1/2 phosphorylation. Pre-treatment with NVP-AEW541 resulted in the inhibition of the FSH-induced ERK 1/2 phosphorylation. Tautomycin did not have any effect (Figure 2, panels a and b). Treatment with FSH increased AKT^{308}/AKT ratio, but by a lesser extent after pre-treatment with NVP-AEW541 and/or tautomycin (Figure 3, panels a and b). FSH also increased AKT^{473}/AKT phosphorylation ratio. Pre-treatment with NVP-AEW541and/or tautomycin hindered the FSH-stimulated AKT^{473} phosphorylation rate (Figure 3, panels c and d). Finally, FSH decreased JNK phosphorylation rate. This effect was not influenced by pre-treatment with NVP-AEW541 and/or tautomycin (Figure 4).

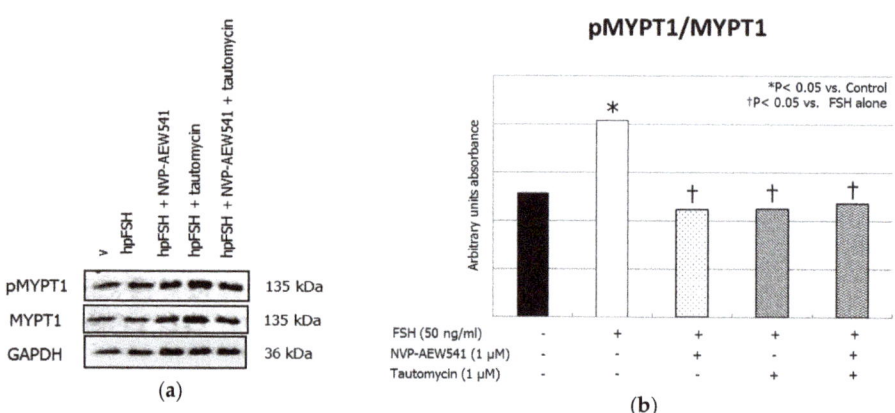

Figure 1. Insulin-like growth factor 1 receptor (IGF1R) is required for the Follicle-stimulating hormone (FSH)-induced myosin-phosphatase 1 (MYPT1) phosphorylation. (**a**) Immunoblots and (**b**) densitometric analysis of phosphorilated myosin-phosphatase 1 (pMYPT1), MYPT1 and Glyceraldehyde-3-Phosphate Dehydrogenase (GADPH) from Sertoli cells alone (control), or incubated with hpFSH alone or pre-treated with the IGF1R inhibitor NVP-AEW541 and/or protein phosphatase 1ß (PP1ß) inhibitor tautomycin and then incubated with hpFSH. Data represent the mean ± standard error of the mean (SEM) (* $p < 0.05$ vs. controls and † $p < 0.05$ vs. FSH treatment alone) (one-way ANOVA) of three independent experiments, each performed in triplicate.

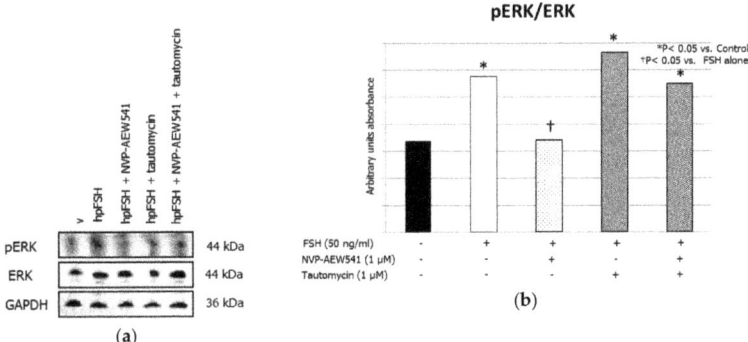

Figure 2. IGF1R is required for the FSH-induced extracellular-signal-regulated kinase (ERK) 1/2 phosphorylation. (**a**) Immunoblots and (**b**) densitometric analysis of the protein bands of pERK1/2, ERK1/2 and Glyceraldehyde-3-Phosphate Dehydrogenase (GADPH) from SCs alone (control) or incubated with hpFSH alone or pre-treated with the IGF1R inhibitor NVP-AEW541 and/or PP1ß inhibitor tautomycin and then incubated with hpFSH. Data represent the mean ± SEM (* $p < 0.05$ vs. controls and † $p < 0.05$ vs. FSH treatment alone) (one-way ANOVA) of three independent experiments, each performed in triplicate.

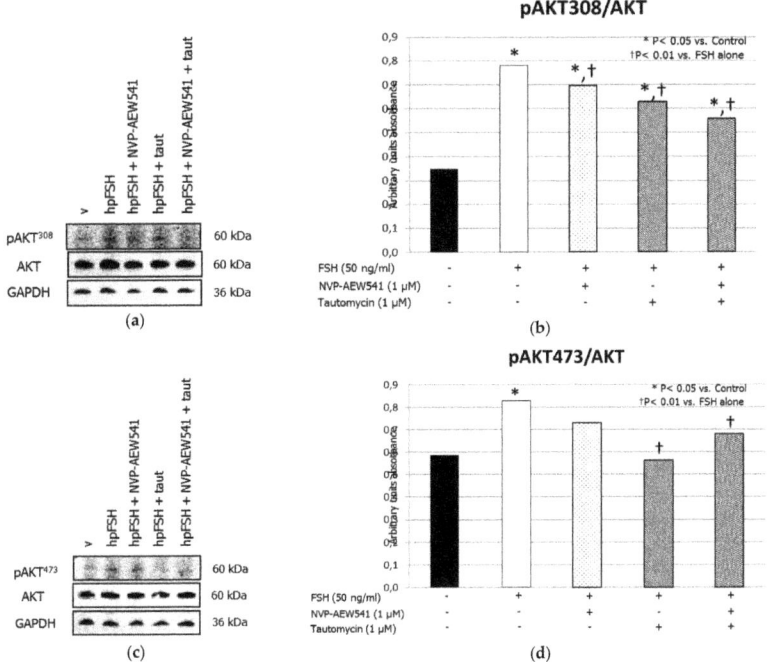

Figure 3. IGF1R is involved in the FSH-induced Protein kinase B (AKT) (Thr308) phosphorylation. (**a**) Immunoblots and (**b**) densitometric analysis of the protein bands of pAKT^{308}, AKT and GADPH and (**c**) Immunoblots and (**d**) densitometric analysis of the protein bands of pAKT^{473}, AKT and GADPH from SCs alone (control), or incubated with hpFSH alone or pre-treated with the IGF1R inhibitor NVP-AEW541 and/or PP1ß inhibitor tautomycin and then incubated with hpFSH. Data represent the mean ± SEM (* $p < 0.05$ vs. control and † $p < 0.01$ vs. FSH treatment alone) (one-way ANOVA) of three independent experiments, each performed in triplicate.

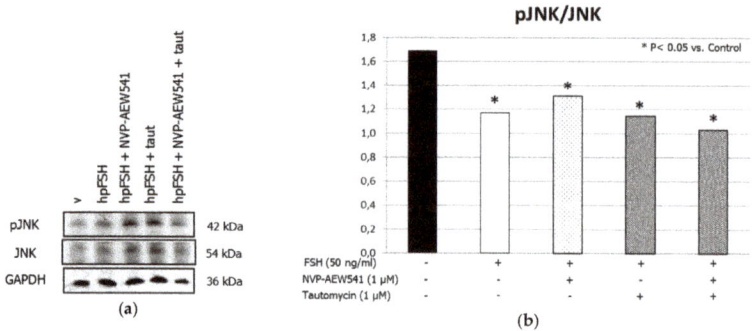

Figure 4. IGF1R does not influence the FSH-induced JNK (Thr18/Tyr185, Thr221/Tyr223) dephosphorylation. (**a**) Immunoblots and (**b**) densitometric analysis of the protein bands of pJNK, JNK and GADPH from SCs alone (control), or incubated with hpFSH alone or pre-treated with the IGF1R inhibitor NVP-AEW541 and/or PP1ß inhibitor tautomycin and then incubated with hpFSH. Data represent the mean ± SEM (* $p < 0.05$ vs. control) (one-way ANOVA) of three independent experiments, each performed in triplicate.

3.2. mRNA Analysis

Treatment with FSH decreased significantly AMH mRNA levels compared to control (−54.7%, $p < 0.01$). The extent of this inhibition was lower in pre-treated cultures (−22.6%, $p < 0.05$ vs. control) (Figure 5, panel a). FSH increased inhibin B mRNA levels compared to control (+487%, $p < 0.01$). These effects were not influenced by pre-treatment with NVP-AEW541 (+501%, $p < 0.01$ vs. control) (Figure 5, panel b). FSH exposure also decreased FSHR mRNA levels compared to control (−59.1%, $p < 0.01$). This was inhibited by NVP-AEW541 pre-treatment (−15%, $p > 0.05$ vs. control) (Figure 5, panel c).

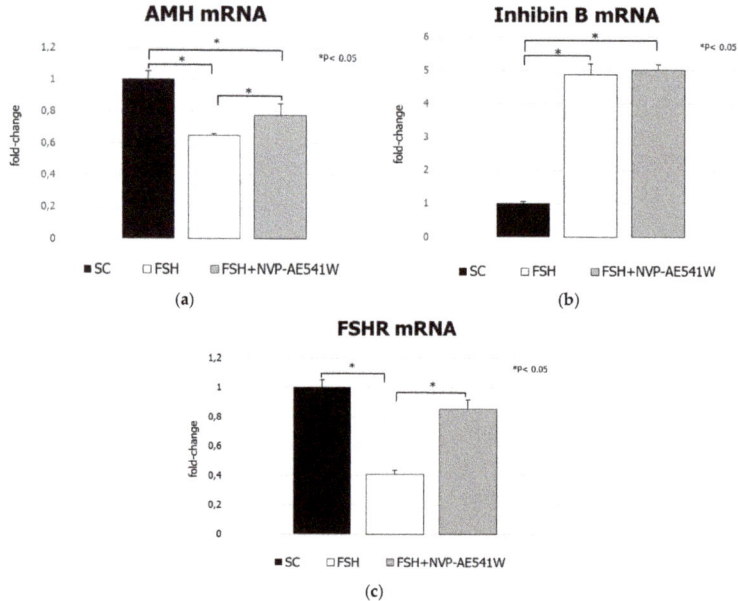

Figure 5. Reverse transcription polymerase chain reaction analysis of (**a**) anti-Müllerian hormone, (**b**) inhibin B and (**c**) FSHR gene expression. Data represent the mean ± SD (* $p < 0.05$ vs. control or FSH treatment) (one-way ANOVA) of three independent experiments, each performed in triplicate.

4. Discussion

We have recently reviewed the effects of the IGF system (mainly IGF1, IGF2 and IGF1R) on testicular differentiation and function in several species including the human one [3]. Altogether, in-vitro evidence suggests that IGF1 and its receptor play a role in basal and FSH-mediated SC or germ cell proliferation [5,10].

Data from mouse granulosa cells have shown the involvement of the IGF1R in FSH signaling. In greater details, IGF1R was required for the FSH-dependent AKT^{308}, AKT^{473}, IRS^{1989} and IGF1RTyr$^{1135/1136}$ phosphorylation [8]. In addition, pre-treatment with tautomycin, a PP1 inhibitor, suppressed the FSH-induced AKT^{308}, AKT^{473}, IRS^{1989} phosphorylation, thus suggesting that the serine/threonine (Ser/Thr) PP1 is necessary for the FSH-mediated IRS1 and AKT phosphorylation. Data from zebrafish confirmed such findings. Indeed, incubation with FSH (promoting type A and B spermatogonia proliferation) increased the IGF3 (a fish-specific member of the IGF family) expression by the PKA and ERK pathways. The FSH-induced proliferation was hindered by the incubation with an IGF3R inhibitor in type A spermatogonia [10].

The results of the present study seem to confirm the existence of an interplay between FSH and IGF1R signaling in SCs. Accordingly, we found that both PP1 and IGF1R inhibition resulted in a lack of FSH-mediated MYPT1 phosphorylation in porcine SCs. Therefore, it may be hypothesized that, similarly to what reported in granulosa cells, IGF1R, IRS1, PP1 and MYPT1 gather together in a molecular complex that requires a conserved tyrosine kinase activity of PP1 and IGF1R to achieve a normal MYPT1 phosphorylation rate under FSH stimulation.

Moreover, in porcine SCs, the FSH-stimulated ERK1/2 phosphorylation occur with an IGF1R-dependent mechanism. PP1 showed to be replaceable for this outcome. Curiously, the double PP1 and IGF1R inhibition did not affect the FSH ability to phosphorylate ERK1/2. In addition, the FSH-dependent AKT phosphorylation was affected by PP1 or IGF1R inhibition. This was expectable since the phosphorylation of AKT reflects the degree of PI3K activation, which in turn is triggered by the IGF1R [19,20].

For the first time, we have also observed that a JNK dephosphorylation occurred after the exposure to FSH. This outcome was not affected by PP1 or IGF1R inhibition. Finally, the FSH-induced downregulation of AMH and FSHR gene expression was IGF1R-mediated. By contrast, IGF1R did not interfere with the FSH-mediated enhancement of inhibin B gene expression.

Porcine SCs have a high degree of similarity with the human ones. Indeed, they have been used in human transplantation experimental protocols for the treatment of patients with type I diabetes mellitus without the need of immunosuppressive therapy [21–23]. Given this similarity, the existence of an interplay between the IGF1R and FSH signaling in human SCs cannot be excluded. According the positive correlation between IGF1 levels and testicular volume in men supports this hypothesis [24]. In addition, the testicular to pubic bone distance, which has been proposed as a marker of testicular post-natal function, has been found to positively correlate with IGF1 in children [25]. The understanding of the role of IGF1 and its receptor on human SC physiology, as well as the possible influence on FSH effects, might help to elucidate some cases of unexplained male infertility. Data on infertile women suggest that this topic deserve further investigation. In fact, a meta-analytic study showed the efficacy of GH administration (which in turn increases IGF1 levels) in combination with gonadotropins in poor responder women undergoing to controlled ovarian hyper-stimulation for assisted reproductive technologies compared to standard therapy [26].

Our results need to be taken with care since the present experimental model does not resemble the complexity of the testicular tissue. Indeed, being an in-vitro study carried out only on SCs, we do not know how the paracrine cross-talk with Leydig cells might impact the SCs responsiveness to FSH in the presence of IGF1R inhibition in vivo. Second, we referred to protocols adopted in granulosa cells for doses and time of incubation, but dose-response analysis of tautomycin, NVP-AEW541 and FSH incubation in SCs are warranted. All these limitations should be taken into consideration in further experimental studies.

5. Conclusions

In conclusion, the results of this study suggest that IGF1R has a role in the modulation of FSH signaling in porcine SCs. The effects of IGF1 on SC physiology deserve further investigation.

Author Contributions: Conceptualization, R.C. (Rossella Cannarella), I.A. and A.E.C.; methodology, C.L., A.A., R.A.C.; software, F.B. and C.B.; validation, G.L.; resources, R.C. (Riccardo Calafiore); data curation, F.M.; writing—original draft preparation, R.C. (Rossella Cannarella); writing—review and editing, R.C. (Rossella Cannarella), S.L.V. and A.E.C.; supervision, S.L.V., F.M. and A.E.C.

Conflicts of Interest: The authors declare no conflict of interest.

References

1. Themmen, A.P.N.; Huhtaniemi, I.T. Mutations of gonadotropins and gonadotropin receptors: Elucidating the physiology and pathophysiology of pituitary-gonadal function. *Endocr. Rev.* **2000**, *21*, 551–583. [CrossRef]
2. Gloaguen, P.; Crépieux, P.; Heitzler, D.; Poupon, A.; Reiter, E. Mapping the follicle-stimulating hormone-induced signaling networks. *Front. Endocrinol.* **2011**, *2*, 45. [CrossRef]
3. Cannarella, R.; Condorelli, R.A.; La Vignera, S.; Calogero, A.E. Effects of the insulin-like growth factor system on testicular differentiation and function: A review of the literature. *Andrology* **2018**, *6*, 3–9. [CrossRef] [PubMed]
4. Nef, S.; Verma-Kurvari, S.; Merenmies, J.; Vassalli, J.D.; Efstratiadis, A.; Accili, D.; Parada, L.F. Testis determination requires insulin receptor family function in mice. *Nature* **2003**, *426*, 291–295. [CrossRef] [PubMed]
5. Pitetti, J.L.; Calvel, P.; Zimmermann, C.; Conne, B.; Papaioannou, M.D.; Aubry, F.; Cederroth, C.R.; Urner, F.; Fumel, B.; Crausaz, M.; et al. An essential role for insulin and IGF1 receptors in regulating sertoli cell proliferation, testis size, and FSH action in mice. *Mol. Endocrinol.* **2013**, *27*, 814–827. [CrossRef] [PubMed]
6. Vanhaesebroeck, B.; Guillermet-Guibert, J.; Graupera, M.; Bilanges, B. The emerging mechanisms of isoform-specific PI3K signalling. *Nat. Rev. Mol. Cell Biol.* **2010**, *11*, 329–341. [CrossRef] [PubMed]
7. Manning, B.D.; Cantley, L.C. AKT/PKB signaling: Navigating downstream. *Cell* **2007**, *129*, 1261–1274. [CrossRef] [PubMed]
8. Law, N.C.; Hunzicker-Dunn, M.E. Insulin Receptor Substrate 1, the Hub Linking Follicle-stimulating Hormone to Phosphatidylinositol 3-Kinase Activation. *J. Biol. Chem.* **2016**, *291*, 4547–4560. [CrossRef] [PubMed]
9. Hunzicker-Dunn, M.E.; Lopez-Biladeau, B.; Law, N.C.; Fiedler, S.E.; Carr, D.W.; Maizels, E.T. PKA and GAB2 play central roles in the FSH signaling pathway to PI3K and AKT in ovarian granulosa cells. *Proc. Natl. Acad. Sci. USA* **2012**, *109*, E2979–E2988. [CrossRef]
10. Nobrega, R.H.; Morais, R.D.; Crespo, D.; de Waal, P.P.; de Franca, L.R.; Schulz, R.W.; Bogerd, J. Fsh stimulates spermatogonial proliferation and differentiation in Zebrafish via Igf3. *Endocrinology* **2015**, *156*, 3804–3817. [CrossRef] [PubMed]
11. Cohen, P.T. Protein phosphatase 1—Targeted in many directions. *J. Cell Sci.* **2002**, *115*, 241–256.
12. Terrak, M.; Kerff, F.; Langsetmo, K.; Tao, T.; Dominguez, R. Structural basis of protein phosphatase 1 regulation. *Nature* **2004**, *429*, 780–784. [CrossRef]
13. Law, N.C.; Donaubauer, E.M.; Zeleznik, A.J.; Hunzicker-Dunn, M. How protein kinase A activates canonical tyrosine kinase signaling pathways to promote granulosa cell differentiation. *Endocrinology* **2017**, *17*, 2043–2051. [CrossRef] [PubMed]
14. Luca, G.; Mancuso, F.; Calvitti, M.; Arato, I.; Falabella, G.; Bufalari, A.; De Monte, V.; Tresoldi, E.; Nastruzzi, C.; Basta, G.; et al. Long-term stability, functional competence, and safety of microencapsulated specific pathogen-free neonatal porcine Sertoli cells: A potential product for cell transplant therapy. *Xenotransplantation* **2015**, *22*, 273–283. [CrossRef] [PubMed]
15. Luca, G.; Arato, I.; Mancuso, F.; Calvitti, M.; Falabella, G.; Murdolo, G.; Basta, G.; Cameron, D.F.; Hansen, B.C.; Fallarino, F.; et al. Xenograft of microencapsulated Sertoli cells restores glucose homeostasis in db/db mice with spontaneous diabetes mellitus. *Xenotransplantation* **2016**, *23*, 429–439. [CrossRef]

16. Mather, J.P.; Philip, D.D. Primary culture of testicular somatic cells. In *Methods for Serum Free Culture of Cells of the Endocrine System*; Barnes, D.W., Sirbasku, D.A., Sato, G.H., Eds.; New York Liss: New York, NY, USA, 1999; pp. 24–45.
17. Arato, I.; Luca, G.; Mancuso, F.; Bellucci, C.; Lilli, C.; Calvitti, M.; Hansen, B.C.; Milardi, D.; Grande, G.; Calafiore, R. An in vitro prototype of a porcine biomimetic testis-like cell culture system: A novel tool for the study of reassembled Sertoli and Leydig cells. *Asian J. Androl.* **2018**, *20*, 160–165.
18. Bradford, M.M. A rapid and sensitive method for the quantitation of microgram quantities of protein utilizing the principle of protein-dye binding. *Anal. Biochem.* **1976**, *72*, 248–254. [CrossRef]
19. Dong, X.C.; Copps, K.D.; Guo, S.; Li, Y.; Kollipara, R.; DePinho, R.A.; White, M.F. Inactivation of hepatic Foxo1 by insulin signaling is required for adaptive nutrient homeostasis and endocrine growth regulation. *Cell Metab.* **2008**, *8*, 65–76. [CrossRef] [PubMed]
20. Copps, K.D.; White, MF. Regulation of insulin sensitivity by serine/threonine phosphorylation of insulin receptor substrate proteins IRS1 and IRS2. *Diabetologia* **2012**, *55*, 2565–2582. [CrossRef]
21. Mital, P.; Kaur, G.; Dufour, J.M. Immunoprotective Sertoli cells: Making allogeneic and xenogeneic transplantation feasible. *Reproduction* **2010**, *139*, 495–504. [CrossRef]
22. Valdes-Gonzalez, R.A.; Dorantes, L.M.; Garibay, G.N.; Bracho-Blanchet, E.; Mendez, A.J.; Davila-Perez, R.; Elliott, R.B.; Teran, L.; White, D.J. Xenotransplantation of porcine neonatal islets of Langerhans and Sertoli cells: A 4-year study. *Eur. J. Endocrinol.* **2005**, *153*, 419–427. [CrossRef]
23. Valdes-Gonzalez, R.A.; White, D.J.; Dorantes, L.M.; Teran, L.; Garibay-Nieto, G.N.; Bracho-Blanchet, E.; Davila-Perez, R.; Evia-Viscarra, L.; Ormsby, C.E.; Ayala-Sumuano, J.T. Three-yr follow-up of a type 1 diabetes mellitus patient with an islet xenotransplant. *Clin. Transplant.* **2007**, *21*, 352–357. [CrossRef] [PubMed]
24. Juul, A.; Bang, P.; Hertel, N.T.; Main, K.; Dalgaard, P.; Jørgensen, K.; Müller, J.; Hall, K.; Skakkebaek, N.E. Serum insulin-like growth factor-I in 1030 healthy children, adolescents, and adults: Relation to age, sex, stage of puberty, testicular size, and body mass index. *J. Clin. Endocrinol. Metab.* **1994**, *78*, 744–752. [PubMed]
25. Koskenniemi, J.J.; Virtanen, H.E.; Wohlfahrt-Veje, C.; Löyttyniemi, E.; Skakkebaek, N.E.; Juul, A.; Andersson, A.M.; Main, K.M.; Toppari, J. Postnatal changes in testicular position are associated with IGF-I and function of Sertoli and Leydig cells. *J. Clin. Endocrinol. Metab.* **2018**, *103*, 1429–1437. [CrossRef] [PubMed]
26. Kyrou, D.; Kolibianakis, E.M.; Venetis, C.A.; Papanikolaou, E.G.; Bontis, J.; Tarlatzis, B.C. How to improve the probability of pregnancy in poor responders undergoing in vitro fertilization: A systematic review and meta-analysis. *Fertil. Steril.* **2009**, *91*, 749–766. [CrossRef] [PubMed]

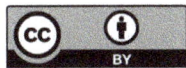

© 2019 by the authors. Licensee MDPI, Basel, Switzerland. This article is an open access article distributed under the terms and conditions of the Creative Commons Attribution (CC BY) license (http://creativecommons.org/licenses/by/4.0/).

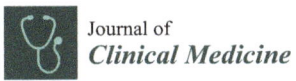 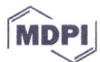

Article

Effects of GH and IGF1 on Basal and FSH-Modulated Porcine Sertoli Cells In-Vitro

Rossella Cannarella [1,*,†], Francesca Mancuso [2,†], Rosita A. Condorelli [1], Iva Arato [2], Laura M. Mongioì [1], Filippo Giacone [1], Cinzia Lilli [2], Catia Bellucci [2], Sandro La Vignera [1], Riccardo Calafiore [3], Giovanni Luca [2,‡] and Aldo E. Calogero [1,‡]

1. Department of Clinical and Experimental Medicine, University of Catania, 95123 Catania, Italy; rosita.condorelli@unict.it (R.A.C.); lauramongioi@hotmail.it (L.M.M.); filippogiacone@yahoo.it (F.G.); sandrolavignera@unict.it (S.L.V.); acaloger@unict.it (A.E.C.)
2. Department of Experimental Medicine, University of Perugia, 06132 Perugia, Italy; francesca.mancuso@unipg.it (F.M.); iva.arato@libero.it (I.A.); cinzia.lilli@unipg.it (C.L.); catia.bellucci@unipg.it (C.B.); Giovanni.luca@unipg.it (G.L.)
3. Department of Medicine, University of Perugia, 06132 Perugia, Italy; riccardo.calafiore@unipg.it
* Correspondence: roxcannarella@gmail.com; Tel.: +39-389-598-6660
† These authors contributed equally to this article.
‡ These authors share the senior authorship of this article.

Received: 28 April 2019; Accepted: 5 June 2019; Published: 6 June 2019

Abstract: Several lines of evidence suggest that insulin-like growth factor 1 (IGF1) is involved in Sertoli cell (SC) proliferation and that its receptor (IGF1R) could mediate follicle-stimulating hormone (FSH) effects. To examine the role of the growth hormone (GH)-IGF1 axis on SC function, we evaluated the effects of GH and IGF1 on basal and FSH-modulated SC proliferation, as well as on anti-Müllerian hormone (AMH) and inhibin B expression and secretion in-vitro. SCs from neonatal pigs were incubated with (1) placebo, (2) 100 nM highly purified urofollitropin (hpFSH), (3) 100 nM recombinant GH (rGH), (4) 100 nM recombinant IGF1 (rIGF1), (5) 100 nM hpFSH plus 100 nM rGH, (6) 100 nM hpFSH plus 100 nM rIGF1, for 48 h. We found that IGF1, but not FSH nor GH, stimulated SC proliferation. Furthermore, an inhibitory effect of FSH, GH and IGF1 on AMH secretion, and a stimulatory role of FSH and IGF1, but not GH, on inhibin B secretion were found. These results suggest that the GH-IGF1 axis influences basal and FSH-modulated SC proliferation and function. We speculate that SC proliferation occurring in childhood might be supported by the increased serum IGF1 levels observed during this period of life.

Keywords: FSH; IGF1; GH; Sertoli cells; AMH

1. Introduction

Sertoli cells (SCs), which represent the major component of the testicular volume in children [1], are mainly committed to sustain spermatogenesis in adulthood. Therefore, an appropriate number of SCs is crucial for male fertility due to structural support, the role they play in the blood–testis barrier and the nourishment that they supply for germ cells (GCs) [2,3].

The insulin/IGF (insulin-like growth factor) signaling pathway has been suggested as one of the major hormonal signals involved in the establishment of a normal-sized cohort of SCs [4]. Pitetti and colleagues provided evidence supporting the importance of both insulin and IGF1 receptors (INSR and IGFR, respectively) in the regulation of SC proliferation, adult testis size and sperm output. Indeed, the weight of the testis of adult mice lacking the *Insr* (SC-*Insr*), the *Igf1r* (SC-*Igf1r*) or both (SC-*Insr;Igf1r*) in SCs is lower compared to wild type ones (weight decrease: 13.6%, 34.6% and 72.4%, respectively) and SCs have a lower proliferation rate during fetal and early neonatal life. This suggests that both insulin and IGF1 are required for the proliferation of immature SCs. Testis from SC-*Igf1r* and SC-*Insr;Igf1r* mice also showed a 38.85% and a 58.71% decrease in epididymal sperm concentration, respectively. Furthermore, in-vivo experiments indicated a role for insulin/IGF signaling in mediating the follicle-stimulating hormone (FSH) effect. Accordingly, FSH administration failed to increase SC number and testis weight in SC-*Insr;Igf1r* mice compared to control animals. Finally, inhibin B gene expression decreased compared to wild type, suggesting that insulin/IGF signaling is needed for FSH-stimulated inhibin B expression. On the contrary, anti-Müllerian hormone (*Amh*) gene expression was not affected [4].

AMH and inhibin B are dimeric glycoproteins secreted by SCs, both belonging to the transforming growth factor-β superfamily. The AMH serum levels reflect the number of immature SCs. Therefore, before puberty, because of the SC immaturity, AMH levels are high, thus representing a possible marker of SC function. At puberty, SCs mature and enter in a quiescence state, therefore, consequently, AMH production decreases and its serum levels decline. The rise in FSH levels, consistent with the beginning of puberty, cause an increase of inhibin B serum levels [1].

The growth hormone (GH) is released by the pituitary gland in a pulsatile manner and it is regulated by the hypothalamic hormones GH-releasing hormone (GHRH) and somatostatin. Despite that IGF1 is commonly believed to be a mediator of GH function, GH receptors (GHR) are expressed in several tissues (e.g., liver, cartilage cells and growth plates of the long bones), suggesting a direct role of GH [5]. GHRs have also been isolated in the testis. This suggests that GH may play a direct role at this level [6]. However, the role of GH on the testicular function has not been investigated.

Recently, an in-vitro pre-pubertal testis-like organ culture system that is highly responsive to human gonadotropins was developed from neonatal porcine testis [7]. This system has been shown to be capable of preserving human sperm viability for up to seven days [8]. It has been proposed as a new model for experimental studies to understand endocrine issues concerning SCs' or Leydig cells' responsiveness to hormone stimuli [7]. Highly-purified FSH (hpFSH) was able to stimulate inhibin B and to inhibit AMH mRNA and protein secretion from SCs in this model [7].

Little is known about the action of GH and IGF1 on porcine SCs. These hormones, which are known to support body growth, are mainly secreted early in mammal life, showing multiple tissue-specific roles [9]. At this time, the testis undergoes physiological changes, consisting of proliferation of immature SC, growth and hormone secretion. These changes precede pubertal SC maturation and the achievement of their final number, as well as the beginning of spermatogenesis [1]. On this account, the aim of this study was to evaluate the in-vitro effects of GH and IGF1 on basal and FSH-modulated SC proliferation, AMH and inhibin B expression and secretion.

2. Experimental Section

2.1. Ethics Statement

This study was carried out in strict compliance with the Guide for the Care and Use of Laboratory Animals of the National Institutes of Health and Perugia University Animal Care. The protocol was approved by the internal Institutional Ethics Committee (Ministry of Health authorization n. 971/2015-PR, 9/14/2015).

2.2. Sertoli Cell Isolation, Culture, Characterization, and Function

SCs were obtained from neonatal pre-pubertal Large White pigs (7–15 days of age) and isolated according to established methods [10]. The fibrous capsule was removed. Then, the testes were finely chopped and digested twice enzymatically, with a mixed solution of trypsin and deoxyribonuclease I (DNase I) in Hanks' balanced salt solution (HBSS; Merck KGaA, Darmstadt, Germany) and collagenase P (Roche Diagnostics S.p.A., Monza, Italy). The tissue pellet was centrifuged, passed through a 500 μm pore stainless steel mesh and then resuspended in glycine to eliminate residual Leydig and peritubular cells [11]. The pellet was then collected and kept in HAM's F12 medium (Euroclone, Milan, Italy) and added with 0.166 nmol L^{-1} retinoic acid (Sigma-Aldrich, Darmstadt, Germany) and 5 mL per 500 mL insulin–transferrin–selenium (ITS, Becton Dickinson cat. no. 354352; Franklin Lakes, NJ, USA) in 95% air/5% CO_2 at 37 °C. Cells were cultured for 3 days. Then, the purity and the functional competence of SC monolayers were assessed, as described elsewhere [6].

2.3. Culture and Treatment

After 3 days of culture, when SC monolayers were confluent, they underwent the following treatments: (1) no treatment; (2) 100 nM highly purified urofollitropin (hpFSH) (Fostimon®, IBSA Farmaceutici Srl, Rome, Italy) for 48 h; (3) 100 nM recombinant growth hormone(rGH) (Saizen 8 mg click.easy, Merck Serono S.p.A.) for 48 h; (4) 100 nM recombinant insulin-like growth factor 1 (r-IGF1) (Sigma Life Science) for 48 h; (5) 100 nM hpFSH and 100 nM rGH for 48 h; (6) 100 nM hpFSH and rIGF1 for 48 h.

2.4. RT-PCR Analysis

Total RNA was extracted and quantified by reading the optical density at 260 nm. In particular, 2.5 µg of total RNA was subjected to reverse transcription (RT, Thermo Scientific, Waltham, MA, USA) to a final volume of 20 µl. The qPCR was performed using 50 ng of the cDNA prepared by RT and a SYBR Green Master Mix (Stratagene, Amsterdam, The Netherlands—Agilent Technology). This was performed in an Mx3000P cycler (Stratagene) using FAM for detection and ROX as the reference dye. The mRNA level of each sample was normalized against β-actin mRNA and expressed as fold change versus the level in untreated control cells.

The following primers were used for Real-time PCR analysis: AMH, forward primers 5′-GCGAACTTAGCGTGGACCTG-3′, revers primers 5′-CTTGGCAGTTGTTGGCTTGATATG-3′; Inhibin B, forward primers 5′-TGGCTGGAGTGACTGGAT-3′, revers primers 5′-CCGTGTGGA AGGATGAGG-3′; FSHR forward primers 5′-TTTCACAGTCGCCCTCTTTCCC-3′, revers primers 5′-TGAGTATAGCAGCCACAGATGACC-3′; actin, forward primers 5′-ATGGTGGGTATGGG TCAGAA-3′, revers primers 5′-CTTCTCCATGTCGTCCCAGT-3′.

2.5. AMH and Inhibin B Secretion Assay

Aliquots of the culture media of treated and untreated SCs were stored at −20 °C for the assessment of AMH (AMH Gen IIELISA, Beckman Coulter; intra-assay CV = 3.89%; inter-assay CV = 5.77%) and inhibin B (Inhibin B Gen II ELISA, Beckman Coulter, Webster, TX, USA; intra-assay CV = 2.81%; inter-assay CV = 4.33%) secretion, as previously described [12].

2.6. Cell Number and Proliferation

After reaching 50%–60% confluence, cells were treated with 0.1 µg/mL colcemid (Sigma-Aldrich no. 10295892001) for 3 h in the incubator [13] and washed with phosphate buffer (PBS). For cell proliferation assay, SC were incubated with 1 µM 5(6)-carboxyfluorescein diacetate N-succinmidyl ester (CFSE, catalog no. 21888, Sigma-Aldrich) in PBS for 8 min and washed with HBSS medium three times. Successively, CFSE-labeled SC were cultured at 37 °C, 5% CO_2 incubator for 48 h following the established protocol of stimulations [hpFSH(100 nM), GH (100 nM), rIGF-1 (100 nM), hpFSH (100 nM) + rGH (100 nM), hpFSH (100 nM) + rIGF1 (100 nM)]. At the end of the stimulation assay, cells were washed with PBS, harvested by tripsinization and then counted using an Automated Cell Counter (Invitrogen, CA, USA) before the flow cytometer analysis [14]. Data acquisition was performed on 20,000 events per tube based on a total (gated alive cells) count of forward and side light scatter at approximately 200–300 events per sec on a BD FAC Sort flow cytometer (BD Biosciences), analyzed using FACS Diva software (BD Biosciences, Franklin Lakes, NJ, USA) and gated on appropriate controls in the different cell populations.

2.7. Statistical Analysis

Results are shown as mean ± SD of three independent experiments, each one performed in triplicate. Data were analyzed for statistical significance by one-way ANOVA, followed by a Tukey post hoc test using SPSS 9.0 for Windows (SPSS Inc., Chicago IL, USA). Significance was accepted for p values lower than 0.05.

3. Results

3.1. Cell Number and Proliferation

Compared to the unexposed control, treatment with hpFSH did not significantly change (1.45 ± 0.07% versus 1.5 ± 0.14%) the percentage of dividing cells. Cell proliferation decreased significantly after incubation with rGH (0.85 ± 0.07% versus 1.5 ± 0.14%, $p < 0.05$). In contrast, rIGF1 exposure significantly increased (1.90 ± 0.14% versus 1.5 ± 0.14%, $p < 0.05$) the percentage of divided cells compared to the control.

Treatment with hpFSH and rGH did not modify the percentage of divided cells (1.15 ± 0.21% versus 1.5 ± 0.14%). This suggests that co-incubation with hpFSH may overcome the inhibitory effect of rGH on cell proliferation. Finally, the simultaneous incubation with hpFSH and rIGF1 significantly increased the percentage of divided cells (2.90 ± 0.21% versus 1.5 ± 0.14%, $p < 0.001$) (Figure 1).

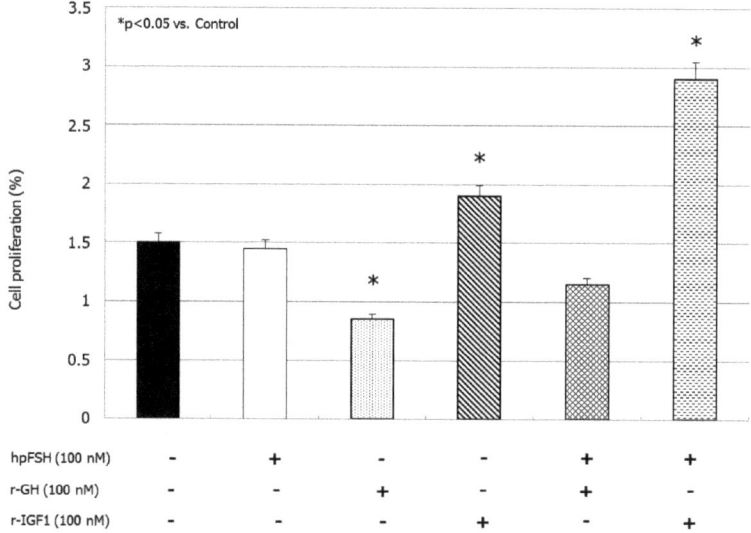

Figure 1. Cell proliferation assay. Data represent the mean ± SD of three independent experiments, each performed in triplicate. (* $p < 0.05$ versus control) (one-way ANOVA). The bars express the percentage of cells with the highest generation number coming from flow cytometric analysis of Sertoli cells stained with CFSE without stimulation after single or combined incubation with hpFSH, rGH or rIGF1.

3.2. FSHR Relative Gene Expression

Treatment with hpFSH or rIGF1 significantly decreased FSHR mRNA levels compared to the control (−41.1% and −46.6%, respectively, $p < 0.0001$). In contrast, rGH significantly increased FSHR mRNA levels (+20.7% versus control, $p < 0.05$).

Co-incubation with hpFSH and rGH significantly decreased FSHR mRNA levels (−31.6%, $p < 0.0001$), suggesting that the stimulatory effects of rGH were counterbalanced by hpFSH. Finally, co-treatment of cell cultures with hpFSH and rIGF1 significantly decreased FSHR mRNA levels compared to the control (−45%, $p < 0.0001$) (Table 1).

Table 1. FSHR relative gene expression in stimulated cultures.

Hormones	Fold Change versus Control (mean ± SD)
hpFSH	0.059 ± 0.06 *
r-GH	1.21 ± 0.12 **
r-IGF1	0.53 ± 0.01 **
hpFSH plus r-GH	0.68 ± 0.03 **
hpFSH plus r-IGF1	0.55 ± 0.00 **

Abbreviations: hpFSH: highly purified follicle-stimulating hormone; r-GH: recombinant growth hormone; r-IGF1: recombinant insulin-like growth factor 1. * $p < 0.05$; ** $p < 0.001$. The mRNA level of each sample was normalized against β-actin mRNA and expressed as fold change versus the level in untreated control cells.

3.3. AMH Gene Expression and AMH Secretion

hpFSH exposure decreased both AMH mRNA levels (−46.1%, $p < 0.005$) and AMH secretion (63.5 ± 2.7 versus 90.1 ± 1.4 μg/cell, $p < 0.0001$) compared to the control. Treatment with rGH reduced AMH secretion (75.5 ± 11.4 versus 90.1 ± 1.4 μg/cell, $p < 0.05$) but did not change the mRNA levels (+0.07%, $p > 0.1$). Incubation with rIGF1 resulted in a significant decrease of the relative gene expression (−60.0%, $p < 0.0001$) levels by the same extent as hpFSH, whereas its inhibitory effect on AMH secretion (44.6 ± 1.4 versus 90.1 ± 1.4 μg/cell, $p < 0.0001$) was stronger than that caused by hpFSH (44.6 ± 1.4 versus 63.5 ± 2.7 μg/cell, $p < 0.005$).

Co-incubation with hpFSH and rGH did not modify the mRNA levels (+0.01%, $p > 0.1$), but it decreased AMH secretion (62.5 ± 1.8 versus 90.1 ± 1.4 μg/cell, $p < 0.0001$) compared to the control. Finally, compared to the control, treatment with rIGF1 plus hpFSH reduced AMH relative gene expression (−50.7%, $p < 0.005$) by the same extent to that obtained with hpFSH alone, however the suppression of AMH secretion (35.6 ± 5.3 versus 90.1 ± 4.4 μg/cell, $p < 0.0001$) was stronger than hpFSH (35.6 ± 5.3 versus 63.5 ± 2.7 μg/cell, $p < 0.0001$) (Figure 2).

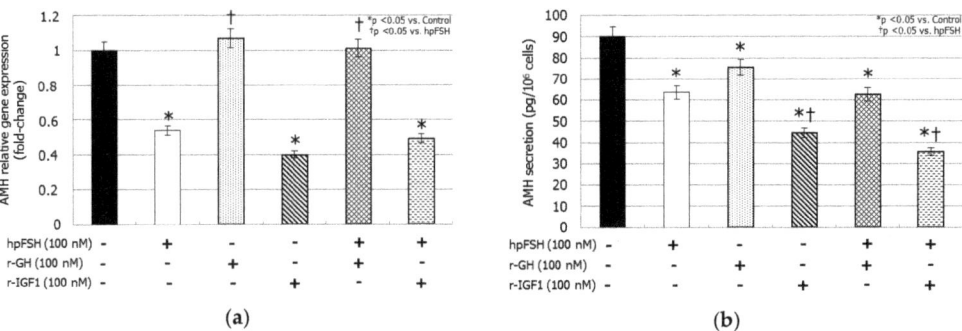

Figure 2. RT-PCR analysis of anti-Müllerian hormone (AMH) gene expression (**a**) and protein secretion (**b**). Data represent the mean ± SD (* $p < 0.05$ versus control and † $p < 0.05$ versus hpFSH treatment) (one-way ANOVA) of three independent experiments, each performed in triplicate.

3.4. Inhibin B Gene Expression and Inhibin B Secretion

Treatment with hpFSH increased both inhibin B mRNA levels (+350%, $p < 0.0001$) and that of the secreted protein (25.52 ± 0.52 versus 2.33 ± 0.75 pg/cell, $p < 0.0001$). In contrast, rGH did not modify inhibin B gene expression (−41.5%, $p > 0.1$) and secretion (1.78 ± 0.20 versus 2.33 ± 0.75 pg/cell, $p > 0.1$). Incubation with rIGF1 resulted in increased inhibin B relative gene expression (+318%, $p < 0.0001$) by the same extent compared to that obtained with hpFSH. rIGF1 also increased the levels of the secreted protein compared to the control (28.03 ± 0.19 versus 2.33 ± 0.75 pg/cell, $p < 0.0001$). The raise of inhibin B levels secreted protein was higher compared to hpFSH (28.03 ± 0.19 versus 25.52 ± 0.52 pg/cell, $p < 0.005$).

Co-incubation with hpFSH and rGH increased gene expression (+410%, $p < 0.0001$) and protein secretion (32.45 ± 0.75 versus 2.33 ± 0.75 pg/cell, $p < 0.0001$) in comparison to the control. The stimulatory effect on protein secretion was stronger compared to that obtained with hpFSH (32.45 ± 0.75 versus 25.52 ± 0.52 pg/cell, $p < 0.0001$). Finally, the co-incubation with hpFSH and rIGF1 increased both mRNA (+295%, $p < 0.0001$) and protein levels (23.73 ± 0.28 versus 2.33 ± 0.75 pg/cell, $p < 0.0001$) compared to the control, with the same extent as hpFSH alone (Figure 3).

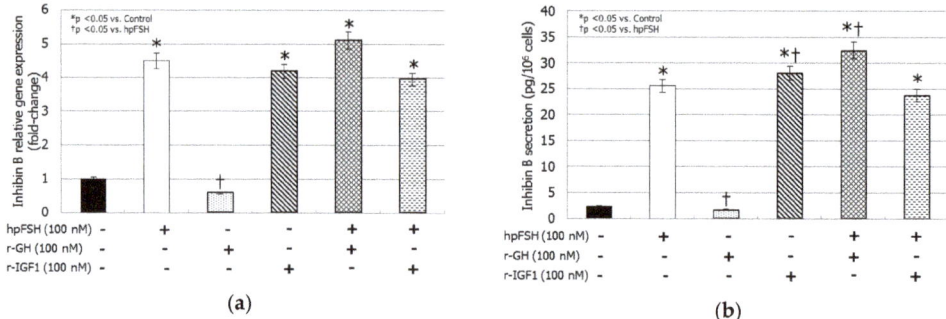

Figure 3. RT-PCR analysis of Inhibin B gene expression (**a**) and protein secretion (**b**). Data represent the mean ± SD (* $p < 0.05$ versus control and † $p < 0.05$ versus hpFSH treatment) (one-way ANOVA) of three independent experiments, each performed in triplicate.

4. Discussion

The major objectives of this study were to assess the role of GH and IGF1 on proliferation and hormonal secretion of SCs from neonatal pigs. During infancy and childhood, testis have erroneously been considered as quiescent due to the low activity of the hypothalamic–gonadotropic axis. However, at this time, SCs are the most numerous, actively proliferating and hormone-secreting cells, and the main cellular component of the testicular volume [14,15]. Different from the hypothalamic–gonadotropic axis, the hypothalamic–somatotropic one is active in childhood [9]. This activity has been regarded as having many tissue-specific functions, being that IGF1R is widely spread in the mammal organism [9], including SCs [16]. Therefore, we sought to investigate whether the hypothalamic–somatotropic axis may influence porcine neonatal testicular SCs. The results of this study showed that both GH and IGF1 were capable of influencing porcine SC proliferation and function, but in a slightly different manner.

Under the experimental conditions used, we found a suppressive effect of GH on SC proliferation. Moreover, it did not affect AMH mRNA but suppressed AMH protein levels. In contrast to FSH, which enhanced inhibin B expression and secretion, GH did not have any significant effect on inhibin B mRNA and protein secretion. The different role of GH and FSH on SC hormone secretion may be further supported by the increased *FSHR* expression in GH-incubated cultures. Furthermore, the FSH-dependent effects on cell proliferation, AMH and inhibin B were not influenced by GH.

To our knowledge, this is the first study investigating the effects of GH on SC proliferation and hormone synthesis. The presence of GH receptors in SCs has already been described [17]. GH has been suggested to play a role in gametogenesis. It was detected in SCs of Japanese eel and its receptors are expressed in germ cells. In a testicular organ culture system, GH stimulation induced germ cell proliferation independently from IGF1 [18]. It was also abundantly detected in secondary spermatocytes and spermatids, myocytes and interstitial cells as well in chicken testis [19]. Furthermore, experimental evidences have shown that the paracrine secretion of GH-releasing hormone (GHRH) from Leydig and germ cells promotes cAMP production in rat SC cultures synergistically with

FSH [18]. GHRH paracrine secretion might also induce GH synthesis in SCs, thus in turn stimulating spermatogenesis. Combining these findings with our results, it appears that SC function is influenced by GH. More in detail, GH seems to influence AMH synthesis in immature SCs and to promote spermatogenesis in mature ones. Whether these effects mainly depend on pituitary- or testis-derived GH is not known. Since human pituitary GH is a ~20 kDa protein, its possible function within the testis would be subordinated by the capacity to cross the testicular blood barrier.

Different from GH, at least at the dosage used in this study, IGF1 enhanced SC proliferation, whereas, surprisingly, FSH alone did not have any effect on this parameter at least at the end of the 48-hour incubation. Similarly to FSH, IGF1 suppressed AMH and increased inhibin B expression and secretion. FSH and IGF1 had similar effects that persisted with the same intensity in co-incubated cultures. Accordingly, *FSHR* was downregulated in cultures incubated with IGF1. In-vitro data indicate a stimulatory effect of IGF1 on germ cell proliferation [16]. Studies in Newt testis [20,21] show a high IGF1 expression in SCs, which is additionally increased after FSH incubation. This brought to hypothesize that FSH-induced spermatogenesis may rely on a paracrine synthesis of IGF1 from SCs [21]. Studies in mutant mice suggest the importance of IGF1 signaling in gonadal male development during embryogenesis [22], as well as in the establishment of a normal-sized SC cohort [4]. Herein, we report the stimulatory effect of IGF1, both alone and in combination with FSH in porcine SCs. Similar results have recently been reported in cultures from pre-pubertal bovine SCs, where the co-incubation with IGF1 and FSH increased cell proliferation and number by ~1.5 fold [23]. Interestingly, and in agreement with such findings, IGF1 serum levels have been found to positively correlate with testicular volume in men [23]. We are not aware of in-vitro studies investigating the effect of IGF1 on AMH and inhibin B secretion from SCs. The similar-to-FSH effects on hormone synthesis are not in contrast with a possible, already suggested IGF1-mediated role on FSH action [16]. The low molecular weight of human IGF1 (~7 kDa) makes it likely that this protein crosses the testicular blood barrier. Hence, a possible pituitary, as well as testis-derived IGF1 role in testicular development and function may be hypothesized.

5. Conclusions

In conclusion, these data indicate that GH and IGF1 are able to influence basal and FSH-modulated SC function. In line with previous evidence [23], we found a stimulatory effect of IGF1, but not of FSH or GH alone, on SC proliferation. Furthermore, both GH, IGF1 and FSH suppressed AMH secretion, whereas IGF1 and FSH, but not GH, stimulated inhibin B synthesis. Wherefore, SC proliferation occurring in childhood may likely be supported by serum IGF1 levels, which are high during this period of life. Since an appropriate number of SCs is needed for spermatogenesis, a lack of IGF1 might compromise SC proliferation and future fertility. The possible relationship between the hypothalamic–somatotropic axis and testis development, AMH and inhibin B serum levels in childhood may, therefore, deserve further investigation.

Author Contributions: Conceptualization, R.C. (Rossella Cannarella); Data curation, I.A. and S.L.V.; Funding acquisition, R.C. (Riccardo Calafiore); Investigation, R.A.C.; Methodology, F.M., F.G., C.L. and C.B.; Project administration, R.C. (Rossella Cannarella), G.L. and A.E.C.; Software, L.M.M.; Supervision, F.M., S.L.V. and A.E.C.; Validation, C.L. and C.B.; Writing—original draft, R.C. (Rossella Cannarella) and F.M.; Writing—review & editing, A.E.C.

Acknowledgments: We thank IBSA Farmaceutici Italia S.r.l. for providing the hpFSH and MERK Serono S.p.a. for providing the rGH used for the experiments.

Conflicts of Interest: The authors declare no conflict of interest.

References

1. Condorelli, R.A.; Cannarella, R.; Calogero, A.E.; La Vignera, S. Evaluation of testicular function in prepubertal children. *Endocrine* **2018**, *62*, 274–280. [CrossRef] [PubMed]
2. Jégou, B. The Sertoli cell. *Baillieres Clin. Endocrinol. Metab.* **1992**, *6*, 273–311. [CrossRef]

3. Mruk, D.D.; Cheng, C.Y. Sertoli-Sertoli and Sertoli-germ cell interactions and their significance in germ cell movement in the seminiferous epithelium during spermatogenesis. *Endocr. Rev.* **2004**, *25*, 747–806. [CrossRef] [PubMed]
4. Pitetti, J.L.; Calvel, P.; Zimmermann, C.; Conne, B.; Papaioannou, M.D.; Aubry, F.; Cederroth, C.R.; Urner, F.; Fumel, B.; Crausaz, M.; et al. An essential role for insulin and IGF1 receptors in regulating sertoli cell proliferation, testis size, and FSH action in mice. *Mol. Endocrinol.* **2013**, *27*, 814–827. [CrossRef] [PubMed]
5. Esposito, S.; Leonardi, A.; Lanciotti, L.; Cofini, M.; Muzi, G.; Penta, L. Vitamin D and growth hormone in children: A review of the current scientific knowledge. *J. Transl. Med.* **2019**, *17*, 87. [CrossRef] [PubMed]
6. Fabbri, A.; Ciocca, D.R.; Ciampani, T.; Wang, J.; Dufau, M.L. Growth hormone-releasing hormone in testicular interstitial and germ cells: Potential paracrine modulation of follicle-stimulating hormone action on Sertoli cell function. *Endocrinology* **1995**, *136*, 2303–2308. [CrossRef]
7. Arato, I.; Luca, G.; Mancuso, F.; Bellucci, C.; Lilli, C.; Calvitti, M.; Hansen, B.C.; Milardi, D.; Grande, G.; Calafiore, R. An in vitro prototype of a porcine biomimetic testis-like cell culture system: A novel tool for the study of reassembled Sertoli and Leydig cells. *Asian J. Androl.* **2018**, *20*, 160–165.
8. Menegazzo, M.; Zuccarello, D.; Luca, G.; Ferlin, A.; Calvitti, M.; Mancuso, F.; Calafiore, R.; Foresta, C. Improvements in human sperm quality by long-term in vitro co-culture with isolated porcine Sertoli cells. *Hum. Reprod.* **2011**, *26*, 2598–2605. [CrossRef]
9. Kineman, R.D.; Del Rio-Moreno, M.; Sarmento-Cabral, A. 40 YEARS of IGF1: Understanding the tissue-specific roles of IGF1/IGF1R in regulating metabolism using the Cre/loxP system. *J. Mol. Endocrinol.* **2018**, *61*, T187–T198. [CrossRef]
10. Luca, G.; Mancuso, F.; Calvitti, M.; Arato, I.; Falabella, G.; Bufalari, A.; De Monte, V.; Tresoldi, E.; Nastruzzi, C.; Basta, G.; et al. Long-term stability, functional competence, and safety of microencapsulated specific pathogen-free neonatal porcine Sertoli cells: A potential product for cell transplant therapy. *Xenotransplantation* **2015**, *22*, 273–283. [CrossRef]
11. Mather, J.P.; Philip, D.D. Primary culture of testicular somatic cells. In *Methods for Serum Free Culture of Cells of the Endocrine System*; Barnes, D.W., Sirbasku, D.A., Sato, G.H., Eds.; New York Liss: New York, NY, USA, 1999; pp. 24–45.
12. Giovagnoli, S.; Mancuso, F.; Vannini, S.; Calvitti, M.; Piroddi, M.; Pietrella, D.; Arato, I.; Falabella, G.; Galli, F.; Moretti, M.; et al. Microparticle-loaded neonatal porcine Sertoli cells for cell-based therapeutic and drug delivery system. *J. Control. Release* **2014**, *192*, 249–261. [CrossRef] [PubMed]
13. Tasiou, V.; Hiber, M.; Steenpass, L. A mouse model for imprinting of the human retinoblastoma gene. *PLoS ONE* **2015**, *10*, e0134672. [CrossRef] [PubMed]
14. Li, B.; Berman, J.; Tang, J.T.; Lin, T.J. The early growth response factor-1 is involved in stem cell factor (SCF)-induced interleukin 13 production by mast cells, but is dispensable for SCF-dependent mast cell growth. *J. Biol. Chem.* **2007**, *282*, 22573–22581. [CrossRef] [PubMed]
15. Valeri, C.; Schteingart, H.F.; Rey, R.A. The prepubertal testis: Biomarkers and functions. *Curr. Opin. Endocrinol. Diabetes Obes.* **2013**, *20*, 224–233. [CrossRef] [PubMed]
16. Cannarella, R.; Condorelli, R.A.; La Vignera, S.; Calogero, A.E. Effects of the insulin-like growth factor system on testicular differentiation and function: A review of the literature. *Andrology* **2018**, *6*, 3–9. [CrossRef] [PubMed]
17. Gomez, J.M.; Loir, M.; Le Gac, F. Growth hormone receptors in testis and liver during the spermatogenetic cycle in rainbow trout (Oncorhynchus mykiss). *Biol. Reprod.* **1998**, *58*, 483–491. [CrossRef] [PubMed]
18. Miura, C.; Shimizu, Y.; Uehara, M.; Ozaki, Y.; Young, G.; Miura, T. Gh is produced by the testis of Japanese eel and stimulates proliferation of spermatogonia. *Reproduction* **2011**, *142*, 869–877. [CrossRef]
19. Nakayama, Y.; Yamamoto, T.; Abé, S.I. IGF-I, IGF-II and insulin promote differentiation of spermatogonia to primary spermatocytes in organ culture of newt testes. *Int. J. Dev. Biol.* **1999**, *43*, 343–347.
20. Yamamoto, T.; Nakayama, Y.; Abé, S.I. Mammalian follicle-stimulating hormone and insulin-like growth factor I (IGF-I) up-regulate IGF-I gene expression in organ culture of newt testis. *Mol. Reprod. Dev.* **2001**, *60*, 56–64. [CrossRef]
21. Pitetti, J.L.; Calvel, P.; Romero, Y.; Conne, B.; Truong, V.; Papaioannou, M.D.; Schaad, O.; Docquier, M.; Herrera, P.L.; Wilhelm, D.; et al. Insulin and IGF1 receptors are essential for XX and XY gonadal differentiation and adrenal development in mice. *PLoS Genet.* **2013**, *9*, e1003160. [CrossRef]

22. Dance, A.; Kastelic, J.; Thundathil, J. A combination of insulin-like growth factor I (IGF-I) and FSH promotes proliferation of prepubertal bovine Sertoli cells isolated and cultured in vitro. *Reprod. Fertil. Dev.* **2017**, *29*, 1635–1641. [CrossRef] [PubMed]
23. Juul, A.; Bang, P.; Hertel, N.T.; Main, K.; Dalgaard, P.; Jørgensen, K.; Müller, J.; Hall, K.; Skakkebaek, N.E. Serum insulin-like growth factor-I in 1030 healthy children, adolescents, and adults: Relation to age, sex, stage of puberty, testicular size, and body mass index. *J. Clin. Endocrinol. Metab.* **1994**, *78*, 744–752. [PubMed]

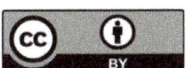

© 2019 by the authors. Licensee MDPI, Basel, Switzerland. This article is an open access article distributed under the terms and conditions of the Creative Commons Attribution (CC BY) license (http://creativecommons.org/licenses/by/4.0/).

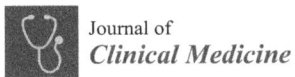

Article

Effects of Insulin on Porcine Neonatal Sertoli Cell Responsiveness to FSH In Vitro

Rossella Cannarella [1,*,†], Iva Arato [2,†], Rosita A. Condorelli [1], Laura M. Mongioì [1], Cinzia Lilli [2], Catia Bellucci [2], Sandro La Vignera [1], Giovanni Luca [2], Francesca Mancuso [2,‡] and Aldo E. Calogero [1,‡]

1. Department of Clinical and Experimental Medicine, University of Catania, 95123 Catania, Italy; rosita.condorelli@unict.it (R.A.C.); lauramongioi@hotmail.it (L.M.M.); sandrolavignera@unict.it (S.L.V.); acaloger@unict.it (A.E.C.)
2. Department of Experimental Medicine, University of Perugia, 06132 Perugia, Italy; iva.arato@libero.it (I.A.); cinzia.lilli@unipg.it (C.L.); catia.bellucci@unipg.it (C.B.); giovanni.luca@unipg.it (G.L.); francesca.mancuso@unipg.it (F.M.)
* Correspondence: roxcannarella@gmail.com; Tel.: +39-389-598-6660
† These authors contributed equally to this article.
‡ These authors share the senior authorship of this article.

Received: 6 May 2019; Accepted: 3 June 2019; Published: 6 June 2019

Abstract: There is ongoing debate as to whether the decline of sperm production in recent times may be related to a parallel increase in the rate of obesity and diabetes. Lower anti-Müllerian hormone (AMH) and inhibin B secretion have been observed in young hyperinsulinemic patients compared to healthy controls, suggesting a Sertoli cell (SC) dysfunction. The pathophysiological mechanisms underlying SC dysfunction in these patients are poorly understood. To the best of our knowledge, no evidence is available on the effects of insulin on SC function. Therefore, this study was undertaken to assess the effects of insulin on basal and follicle-stimulating hormone (FSH)-stimulated SC function in vitro. To accomplish this, we evaluated the expression of *AMH*, *inhibin B* and *FSHR* genes, the secretion of AMH and inhibin B and the phosphorylation of AKT473 and SC proliferation on neonatal porcine SC after incubation with FSH and/or insulin. We found that similar to FSH, the expression and secretion of AMH is suppressed by insulin. Co-incubation with FSH and insulin decreased AMH secretion significantly more than with FSH alone. Insulin had no effect on the expression and secretion of the *inhibin B* gene, but co-incubation with FSH and insulin had a lower effect on inhibin B secretion than that found with FSH alone. FSH and/or insulin increased AKT473 phosphorylation and SC proliferation. In conclusion, the results of this study showed that insulin modulates SC function. We hypothesize that hyperinsulinemia may therefore influence testicular function even before puberty begins. Therefore, particular care should be taken to avoid the onset of hyperinsulinemia in children to prevent a future deleterious effect on fertility.

Keywords: FSH; insulin; Sertoli cells; AMH; inhibin B

---

1. Introduction

Sertoli cells (SCs), the only somatic constituent of the testicular seminiferous epithelium, are mainly involved in supporting spermatogenesis. In particular, they provide structural support to germ cells (GCs), constitute the blood–testicular barrier, assist the movement of GCs within the seminiferous epithelium and guide the maturation of GCs through secretion products. Notably, they support a finite number of GCs [1,2].

Anti-Müllerian hormone (AMH) and inhibin B are dimeric glycoproteins secreted by SCs; both of these hormones belong to the transforming growth factor-β superfamily. Immature and actively proliferating SCs may be found in the testis until puberty. At this stage, the testis is mainly made up of AMH-secreting SCs. The overall number of SCs is known to impact testicular volume. The amount of AMH secreted reflects SC immaturity. When puberty begins, SCs pass to a state of maturity and quiescence. As a result, serum AMH levels decrease while those of inhibin B increase in a follicle-stimulating hormone (FSH)-dependent manner. Concomitant with the onset of spermatogenesis, the testicular volume increases and GCs become the predominant testicular component (for review, see [3,4]).

FSH acts through a G-protein-coupled (GPCR) receptor (FSHR) in SCs. Once stimulated by FSH, as for many GPCRs, the FSHR triggers the Gαs, which activates the adenylate cyclase, resulting in increased intracellular cAMP levels. The latter leads to protein kinase A (PKA) activation [5], which in turn triggers the following major signaling pathways: the phosphoinositide 3-kinase (PI3K)/AKT pathway and the mitogen-activated protein kinase (MAPK) pathway [6,7]. The first is committed to preventing apoptosis, cell proliferation and glucose transport. It is activated in an insulin-like growth factor 1 receptor (IGF1R)-dependent manner [7]. The MAPK pathways, including ERK1/2 and JNK, regulate cell proliferation, differentiation and apoptosis [6]. Both of these pathways are activated by insulin and the insulin-like growth factor (IGF) family [8].

Insulin receptor (INSR) and IGF1R are expressed in SCs [9] and have been found to play a role in adrenal and testis differentiation [6]. The SC-selective knock-out for *INSR* and/or *IGF1R* genes has been shown to have a negative effect on testicular volume in mice [10]. In particular, the SC-INSR knock-out was associated with a 13.6% testis weight decrease, the SC-IGF1R knock-out with a 34.6% decrease and the combined SC-INSR/IGF1R knock-out with a 72.4% testis weight reduction [10], thus suggesting a role for both receptors in SC proliferation.

There is ongoing debate as to whether the decline of sperm production in recent times [11] is related to the parallel increase in the rate of obesity and diabetes [12]. Some evidence points to a possible negative impact of hyperinsulinemia on SC function before puberty, since lower AMH and inhibin B levels have been found in young obese patients compared to normal weight controls [13–15]. However, studies on the possible mechanism(s) are lacking and, therefore, no data are available to date on the effect of insulin on SC function.

As cultures of SCs from pre-pubertal porcine testes have been developed to reproduce an in vitro reliable prototype of pre-pubertal human testicular tissue [16], the purpose of this study was to evaluate the effects of insulin on both basal and FSH-stimulated SC function in this model to better understand the rationale of the results reported in humans [13–15]. To accomplish this, we evaluated the expression of *AMH*, *inhibin B* and *FSHR* genes, the secretion of AMH and inhibin B, the phosphorylation of AKT473 and the proliferation of SC after incubation with insulin.

2. Experimental Section

2.1. Ethics Statement

This study was conducted in strict compliance with the Guide for the Care and Use of Laboratory Animals of the National Institutes of Health and Perugia University Animal Care. The protocol was approved by the internal Institutional Ethic Committee (Ministry of Health authorization n. 971/2015-PR, 9/14/2015).

2.2. Sertoli Cell Isolation, Culture, Characterization and Function

SCs, obtained from neonatal prepubertal Large White pigs, 7–15 days of age, were isolated according to established methods, with slight modifications [17]. Briefly, after removing the fibrous capsule, the testes were finely chopped and digested twice enzymatically with a mixed solution of trypsin and deoxyribonuclease I (DNase I) in Hanks' balanced salt solution (HBSS; Merck KGaA,

Darmstadt, Germany) and collagenase P (Roche Diagnostics S.p.A., Monza, Italy). The tissue pellet was centrifuged through a 500 µm pore stainless steel mesh. It was then re-suspended in glycine to eliminate residual Leydig and peritubular cells [18]. The resulting pellet was collected and maintained in HAM's F12 medium (Euroclone, Milan, Italy), supplemented with 0.166 nmol l−1 retinoic acid, (Sigma-Aldrich, Darmstadt, Germany) and 5 mL per 500 mL insulin-transferrin-selenium (Becton Dickinson cat. no. 354352; Franklin Lakes, NJ, USA) in 95% air/5% CO_2 at 37 °C. After 3 days in culture, the purity and the functional competence of SC monolayers were determined according to previously established methods [16].

2.3. Culture and Treatment

When SC monolayers were confluent (after 3 days of culture), they were incubated for 48 h as follows: (1) placebo; (2) 100 nM highly purified urofollitropin (hpFSH) (Fostimon®, IBSA Farmaceutici Srl, Rome, Italy); (3) 100 nM recombinant insulin (rInsulin) (Humalog, Eli Lilly Srl, Florence, Italy); (4) 100 nM hpFSH and 100 nM rInsulin.

2.4. RT-PCR Analysis

Total RNA was extracted with Trizol® Reagent (Life Techologies, Waltham, MA, USA) according to the manufacturer's instructions. RNA concentration and purity were determined using Biophotometer Eppendorf. cDNA reverse transcription was carried out for each sample using a cDNA synthesis kit (Thermo Scientific Maxima First Strand cDNA Synthesis Kit for RT-qPCR), according to the manufacturer's instruction.

The qPCR was performed using 50 ng of the cDNA prepared by RT and a SYBR Green Master Mix (Stratagene, Amsterdam, The Netherlands) (Agilent Technology), using the following primers: AMH, forward primers 5′-GCGAACTTAGCGTGGACCTG-3′, reverse primers 5′-CTTGGCAGTTGTT GGCTTGATATG-3′; inhibin B, forward primers 5′-TGGCTGGAGTGACTGGAT -3′, reverse primers 5′-CCGTGTGGAAGGATGAGG-3′; FSHR forward primers 5′-TTTCACAGTCGCCCTCTTTCCC-3′, reverse primers 5′-TGAGTATAGCAGCCACAGATGACC-3′; actin, forward primers 5′-ATGGTGGGT ATGGGTCAGAA-3′, reverse primers 5′-CTTCTCCATGTCGTCCCAGT-3′. qPCR was performed in an Mx3000P cycler (Stratagene), using FAM for detection and ROX as the reference dye.

2.5. AMH and Inhibin B Secretion Assay

Aliquots of the culture media of treated and untreated SCs were collected and stored at −20 °C for the assessment of AMH (AMH Gen II ELISA, Beckman Coulter, Webster, TX, USA) (intra-assay CV = 3.9%; inter-assay CV = 5.8%) and inhibin B (inhibin B Gen II ELISA, Beckman Coulter, Webster, TX, USA) (intra-assay CV = 2.8%; inter-assay CV = 4.3%) concentrations as previously described [19].

2.6. Western Blot (WB) Analysis

At the end of the incubation period, total cell lysates were collected in a radioimmunoprecipitation assay (RIPA) lysis buffer (Santa Cruz Biotechnology Inc., Santa Cruz, CA, USA). The mixture was centrifuged at 1000× *g* (Eppendorf, Hauppauge, NY, USA) for 10 min, the supernatant was collected and total protein content was measured by the Bradford method [20]. Sample aliquots were stored at −20 °C for Western blot (WB) analysis. The cell extracts were separated by 4–12% SDS-PAGE and equal amounts of protein (70 µg protein/lane) were run and blotted on nitrocellulose membranes (BioRad, Hercules, CA, USA). The membranes were incubated overnight in a buffer containing 10 mM TRIS, 0.5 M NaCl, 1% (*v/v*) Tween 20 (Sigma-Aldrich), rabbit anti-phospho-AKT (Ser473) (dilution factor 1:1000) (Cell Signaling, Danvers, MA, USA), rabbit anti-AKT (dilution factor 1:1000) (Cell Signaling) and mouse anti- Glyceraldehyde 3-phosphate dehydrogenase (GADPH) (6C5):sc-32233 (dilution factor 1:200) (Santa Cruz, Biotechnology, CA, USA) primary antibodies. Primary antibody binding was then detected by incubating the membranes for an additional 60 min in a buffer containing horseradish peroxidase conjugated anti-rabbit (Sigma-Aldrich) (dilution factor, 1:5000) and/or anti-mouse (Santa Cruz Biotechnology Inc.) (dilution factor, 1:5000) IgG secondary antibodies. The bands were detected by enhanced chemiluminescence.

2.7. Cell Number and Proliferation

After reaching 50 to 60% confluence, cells were incubated with 0.1 µg/mL colcemid (Sigma-Aldrich, St. Louis, MO, USA) for 3 h [21]. Afterwards they were washed with phosphate buffer (PBS, Lonza, Basel, Switzerland) before the evaluation of the proliferation. For cell proliferation assay, SCs were incubated with 1 µM 5(6)-carboxyfluorescein diacetate N-succinmidyl ester (CFSE) (Sigma-Aldrich, MO, USA) in PBS for 8 min, and then washed with HBSS medium (Lonza, Basel, Switzerland) three times. CFSE-labeled SCs were then cultured at 37 °C and incubated in 5% CO_2 for 48 h with hpFSH (100 nM) and/or insulin (100 nM). At the end of the stimulation assay, cells were washed with PBS, harvested by tripsinization and counted using an Automated Cell Counter (Invitrogen, Carlsbad, CA, USA) before flow cytometer analysis [22]. Data acquisition was performed on 20,000 events per tube based on a total (gated alive cells) count of forward and side light scatter at approximately 200–300 events per second on a BD FACS ortflow cytometer (BD Biosciences, Franklin Lakes, NJ, USA), analyzed using FACS Diva software (4.0 BD Biosciences, Franklin Lakes, NJ, USA) and gated on appropriate controls in the different cell populations.

2.8. Statistical Analysis

Results are shown as the mean ± SEM of three independent experiments, each one performed in triplicate. The average value from the triplicates of each cell culture was used for the statistical analysis. Data were analyzed for statistical significance by one-way ANOVA, followed by the Tukey post-hoc test using SPSS 22.0 for Windows (SPSS Inc., Chicago, IL, USA). A statistically significant difference was accepted when the p value was lower than 0.05.

3. Results

3.1. RT-PCR Analysis

Compared with the untreated control, *AMH* gene expression was significantly downregulated by hpFSH, rInsulin and hpFSH plus rInsulin ($p < 0.05$ vs. control) (Figure 1A). Differences in the mRNA levels of AMH were −46.1, −48.1 and −37.0%, respectively.

Compared with the untreated control, *inhibin B* gene expression was significantly upregulated by hpFSH. The co-incubation with hpFSH plus rInsulin did not significantly affect the stimulatory effect of hpFSH alone (Figure 1B). Differences in the mRNA of inhibin B were +350% ($p < 0.0001$) with hpFSH and +279% ($p < 0.0001$) with hpFSH plus rInsulin. Incubation with rInsulin did not have a significant effect on inhibin B mRNA levels compared with untreated control. Compared with hpFSH stimulation, *inhibin B* gene expression was significantly downregulated by rInsulin (−89.4%; $p < 0.0001$) and a trend for lower levels was found after incubation with hpFSH plus rInsulin (−15.8%; $p = 0.05$).

Finally, compared with the untreated control, *FSHR* gene expression decreased significantly after incubation with hpFSH and/or rInsulin ($p < 0.05$ vs. control) (Figure 1C). Differences in the mRNA levels of rFSH were −41.1, −28.2 and −22.5%, respectively. The co-incubation with rInsulin did not change the decrease of *FSHR* gene expression significantly.

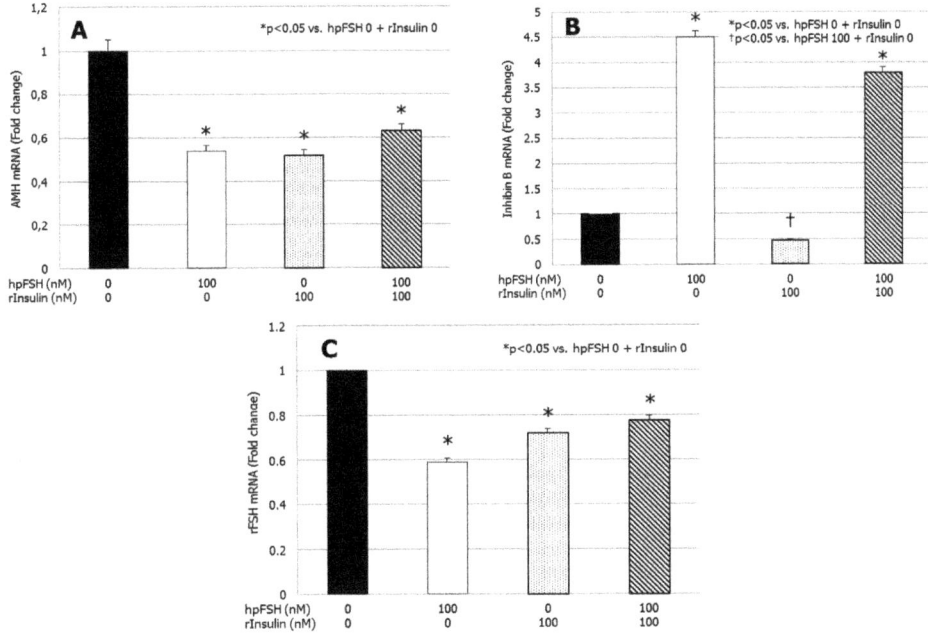

Figure 1. RT-PCR analysis of (**A**) *anti-Müllerian hormone* (*AMH*), (**B**) *inhibin B* and (**C**) *FSHR* gene expression. Data represent the mean ± SEM of three independent experiments, each performed in triplicate. * $p < 0.05$ vs. control; † $p < 0.05$ vs. highly purified urofollitropin (hpFSH) (one-way ANOVA).

3.2. AMH and Inhibin B Secretion

Figure 2A shows a significant decrease of AMH secretion after exposure to hpFSH (63.5 ± 2.7 vs. 90.1 ± 1.4 µg/cell, $p < 0.0001$), rInsulin (52.8 ± 0.6 vs. 90.1 ± 1.4 µg/cell, $p < 0.0001$) and hpFSH plus rInsulin (47.1 ± 0.6 vs. 90.1 ± 4.4 µg/cell, $p < 0.0001$) compared to the untreated control. The co-incubation with hpFSH and rInsulin suppressed AMH secretion significantly compared to that found with hpFSH alone (47.1 ± 0.6 vs. 63.5 ± 2.7 µg/cell, $p < 0.05$). AMH secretion did not differ significantly between hpFSH or rInsulin alone.

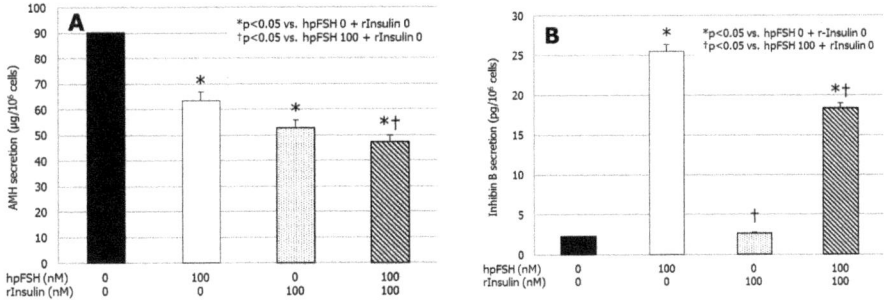

Figure 2. Secretion of (**A**) anti-Müllerian hormone (AMH) and (**B**) inhibin B. Data represent the mean ± SEM of three independent experiments, each performed in triplicate. * $p < 0.05$ vs. control; † $p < 0.05$ vs. hpFSH (one-way ANOVA).

Figure 2B shows a significantly higher secretion of inhibin B after hpFSH (25.52 ± 0.52 vs. 2.3 ± 0.8 pg/cell, $p < 0.0001$) and hpFSH plus rInsulin (18.4 ± 0.3 vs. 2.3 ± 0.8 pg/cell, $p < 0.0001$) incubation compared to the untreated control. Treatment with rInsulin did not change inhibin B secretion significantly compared to the untreated control (2.6 ± 1.3 vs. 2.3 ± 0.8 pg/cell, $p = 0.99$). Compared to hpFSH alone, the co-incubation with hpFSH and rInsulin significantly decreased the secretion of inhibin B (18.4 ± 0.3 vs. 25.5 ± 0.5 pg/cell, $p < 0.0001$).

3.3. Western Blot (WB) Analysis

WB analysis showed that incubation with hpFSH (0.868 ± 0.07; $p < 0.001$), rInsulin (0.928 ± 0.04; $p < 0.001$) or hpFSH plus rInsulin (0.632 ± 0.04; $p < 0.01$) significantly increased AKT phosphorylation compared to the unexposed control (0.511 ± 0.06). Compared to the hpFSH-treated sample, the levels of AKT phosphorylation after hpFSH plus rInsulin exposure were significantly lower (0.632 ± 0.04 vs. 0.868 ± 0.07, $p < 0.01$) (Figure 3).

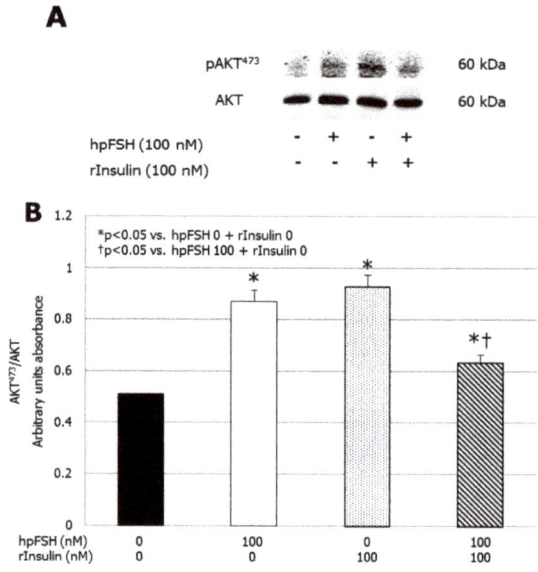

Figure 3. (**A**) Immunoblots and (**B**) densitometric analysis of the protein bands of pAKT473 and AKT of unexposed samples (control) and after incubation with hpFSH, rInsulin or hpFSH plus rInsulin. Data represent the mean ± SEM of three independent experiments, each performed in triplicate. * $p < 0.05$ vs. control; † $p < 0.05$ vs. hpFSH (one-way ANOVA).

3.4. Cell Number and Proliferation

Compared to the untreated control, the percentage of divided cells did not differ after exposure to hpFSH (1.5 ± 0.7 vs. 1.5 ± 0.1%, $p > 0.99$). Treatment with rInsulin or hpFSH plus rInsulin significantly increased the percentage of divided cells compared to the control (2.1 ± 0.1 vs. 1.5 ± 0.1%, $p < 0.05$ and 2.8 ± 0.0 vs. 1.5 ± 0.1%, $p < 0.001$) (Figures 4 and 5).

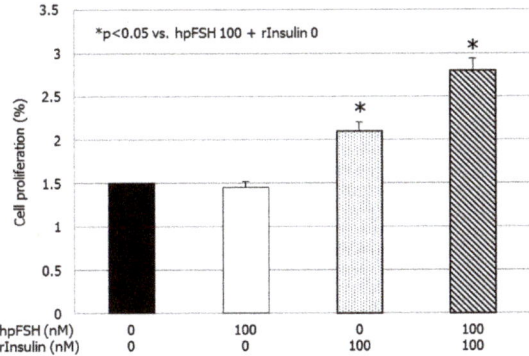

Figure 4. Cell proliferation assay. Data represent the mean ± SEM of three independent experiments, each performed in triplicate. * $p < 0.05$ vs. control (one-way ANOVA).

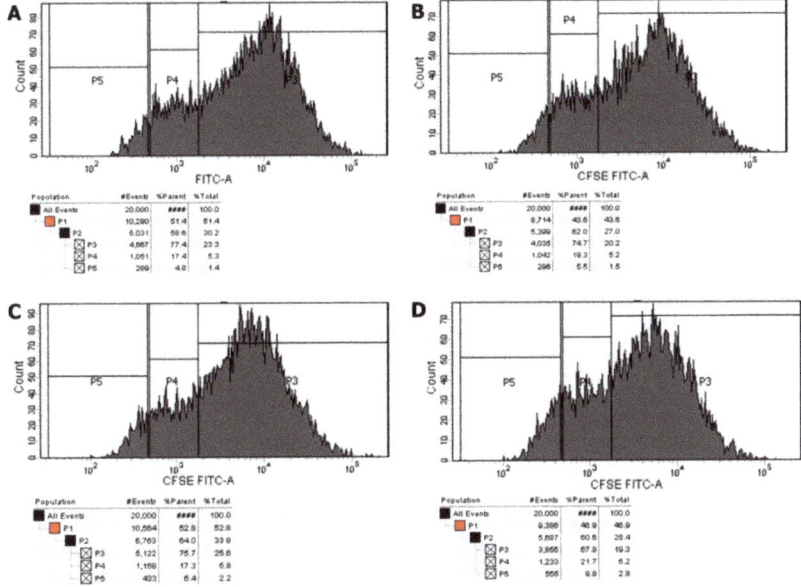

Figure 5. Flow cytometric analysis. Flow cytometric analysis of Sertoli cells stained with carboxyfluorescein diacetate N-succinmidyl ester (CFSE) without stimulation (**A**), and after incubation with hpFSH (**B**), rInsulin (**C**), hpFSH and rInsulin (**D**). Gray peaks represent successive generations.

4. Discussion

Metabolic diseases (e.g., obesity, insulin resistance, diabetes mellitus) have long been considered possible etiopathogenetic causes of male infertility [23–25]. However, the pathophysiological mechanisms are still elusive. To the best of our knowledge, no evidence is available on the effects of insulin on SC function. Our data suggest that SCs are responsive to insulin, which influences SC secretion patterns and proliferation. Similar to FSH, insulin downregulated AMH expression and secretion. Co-incubation with FSH and insulin lowered AMH secretion more than FSH alone. Furthermore, we found that insulin did not influence inhibin B expression and secretion, but FSH plus insulin lessened the effects of FSH, since inhibin B levels were lower in co-incubated cultures compared with those found in cultures stimulated with FSH alone.

These findings are consistent with the data reported in humans. An observational study carried out in pre-pubertal boys aged 5–9 years and young adult men aged 18–24 years found lower levels of inhibin B in obese (body mass index (BMI) > 30 kg/m^2) patients compared to the normal weight (BMI < 25 kg/m^2) controls. No difference was found in pre-pubertal boys. Unfortunately, despite the occurrence of hyperinsulinemia that might be supposed in the obese patients, insulin serum levels were not measured or reported [13].

More recently, a study involving 121 obese and 38 lean adolescents in the pubertal phase (Tanner stage ≥ 2) found lower levels of AMH and inhibin B in obese patients compared to controls. Obese patients also had higher levels of insulin whereas no significant differences in FSH levels were found [14]. It is noteworthy that the longitudinal study of the Western Australian Pregnancy Cohort (Raine), involving male children born in 1989–1991 followed from birth until the age of 20 years, has shown that patients with insulin resistance (Homeostatic Model Assessment of Insulin Resistance (HOMA) > 4), probably being hyperinsulinemics, had lower inhibin B and higher FSH levels at the age of 17–20 years, even after adjusting for age, body mass index, abstinence, history of cryptorchidism, varicocele, cigarette smoking, alcohol consumption and drugs (Hart et al., 2019). Low levels of AMH and inhibin B have been considered as biochemical signs of SC dysfunction in childhood and adolescence. Therefore, their measurement can help in the early identification of an isolated primary testicular tubulopathy, intercepting patients at risk of future infertility [4].

Altogether, these data highlight the negative impact of metabolic diseases on SC function, both before puberty, when only AMH secretion is affected, and after puberty, when inhibin B secretion is also impaired [13–15]. This is consistent with the results of the current study. SCs not exposed to FSH resemble a condition that occurs in pre-pubertal testes that are not physiologically exposed to FSH. At this time, hyperinsulinemia only affects AMH levels and does not have any effect on inhibin B [13,14]. Cells incubated with FSH provide data on how SCs can behave in the pubertal phase when they begin to be under the influence of FSH. In this phase of life, as suggested by human studies [13,14] and confirmed by the present in vitro data, hyperinsulinemia suppresses FSH-stimulated inhibin B secretion.

In addition, Hart and colleagues [15] observed lower sperm production in insulin-resistant 20 year old patients than in age-matched lean controls. Taken together, these data suggest a causal link between the increased prevalence of metabolic diseases [12] and the decline in sperm production [11]. Therefore, weight loss should be encouraged in obese children to preserve their future fertility.

The results of the present study suggest that a cross-talk between FSH and insulin might exist in porcine SCs. FSH has recently been shown to enhance myosin-phosphatase 1 (MYPT1), ERK 1/2, AKT^{308}, AKT^{473} and to decrease JNK phosphorylation rates. These effects were partially or totally hindered by pre-treatment with the insulin-like growth factor 1 receptor (IGF1R) inhibitor NVP-AEW541, thus suggesting a role for IGF1R in FSH signaling [7]. Studies carried out in granulosa cells supported these data [26] and further indicated that insulin-receptor substrate 1 (IRS1) might be the hub linking FSHR, belonging to the G protein-coupled receptors (GPCRs), and IGF1R, which is a tyrosine kinase receptor [27]. IRS1 is involved in the insulin receptor signaling and is known to play a role in insulin sensitivity as insulin-resistant animal models show higher phosphorylation rates of this protein compared to healthy ones [28]. Taking all this into account, the cross-talk between FSH and insulin might involve IRS1, especially in case of insulin resistance, but this needs to be elucidated. Taking into account the findings of *FSHR* gene expression, we hypothesize that insulin might interfere with FSH signaling and action (which is consistent with data from insulin-resistant or obese children and adolescents) through *FSHR* downregulation. However, further studies analyzing the FSH and insulin receptors signaling pathway in SCs and the FSHR protein expression after hormone incubation are warranted to better clarify this topic.

We found an increase in AKT phosphorylation in SCs incubated with insulin. As mentioned before, the MAPK pathway is committed to cell proliferation [8]. As a result, and in contrast to FSH, insulin increased SC proliferation. This is in line with data on SC-selective INSR knock-out mice that have a lower testicular volume than that found in the wild type [10]. Data from a chicken model confirm the stimulating role of insulin on SC cultures [29]. These authors also reported a lack of AKT phosphorylation and SC proliferation in metformin-exposed SC cultures from insulin-resistant chickens [29]. The negative impact of metformin on SC proliferation was also confirmed in rats [30] and, consequently, the in vivo administration of metformin to pregnant mice caused the birth of pups with low testicular volumes, which was associated with a lower number of SCs [31]. Taken together, these data discourage metformin administration in obese boys, where SC is still actively proliferating [4]. The mechanisms through which this drug exerts such an anti-proliferative effect on SCs deserves further investigation.

Since the in vitro experimental model used in this study does not resemble the complexity of in vivo testicular tissue, the present findings should be taken with caution. We used a pure culture of SCs, and possible different in vivo responses due to the paracrine cross-talk between SC and Leydig cells cannot be excluded. Therefore, in vivo studies are needed to confirm such findings.

5. Conclusions

In conclusion, to our knowledge, this is the first study showing the influence of insulin on the secretion of AMH and inhibin B both basally and in response to FSH in primary porcine SC cultures. Under basal conditions, insulin suppressed AMH release but had no effect on inhibin B secretion. In addition, insulin influenced the SC responsiveness to FSH by lowering the amount of AMH and inhibin B compared to the cultures stimulated with FSH alone. Finally, insulin increased SC proliferation, confirming the results on mice with an SC-selective *INSR* gene knock-out [10]. These results could provide the rationale for the lower AMH and inhibin B levels found in obese or insulin-resistant boys and young men compared to normal weight controls [13–15], thus highlighting the importance of assessing testicular function in pre-pubertal obese children [10].

Author Contributions: Conceptualization, R.C. and A.E.C.; Data curation, C.L. and C.B.; Funding acquisition, S.L.V. and G.L.; Investigation, I.A. and R.A.C.; Methodology, R.A.C. and L.M.M.; Project administration, R.C. and A.E.C.; Resources, G.L.; Supervision, S.L.V. and F.M.; Validation, C.L. and C.B.; Writing—Original draft, R.C., I.A. and F.M.; Writing—Review and editing, A.E.C.

Acknowledgments: We thank IBSA Farmaceutici Italia S.r.l. for providing the hpFSH used for the experiments.

Conflicts of Interest: The authors declare no conflict of interest.

References

1. Jégou, B. The sertoli cell. *Baillieres Clin. Endocrinol. Metab.* **1992**, *6*, 273–311. [CrossRef]
2. Mruk, D.D.; Cheng, C.Y. Sertoli-sertoli and sertoli-germ cell interactions and their significance in germ cell movement in the seminiferous epithelium during spermatogenesis. *Endocr. Rev.* **2004**, *25*, 747–806. [CrossRef] [PubMed]
3. Edelsztein, N.Y.; Grinspon, R.P.; Schteingart, H.F.; Rey, R.A. Anti-müllerian hormone as a marker of steroid and gonadotropin action in the testis of children and adolescents with disorders of the gonadal axis. *Int. J. Pediatr. Endocrinol.* **2016**, *2016*, 20. [CrossRef] [PubMed]
4. Condorelli, R.A.; Cannarella, R.; Calogero, A.E.; La Vignera, S. Evaluation of testicular function in prepubertal children. *Endocrine* **2018**, *62*, 274–280. [CrossRef] [PubMed]
5. Gloaguen, P.; Crépieux, P.; Heitzler, D.; Poupon, A.; Reiter, E. Mapping the follicle-stimulating hormone-induced signaling networks. *Front. Endocrinol. (Lausanne)* **2011**, *2*, 45. [CrossRef] [PubMed]
6. Pitetti, J.L.; Calvel, P.; Romero, Y.; Conne, B.; Truong, V.; Papaioannou, M.D.; Schaad, O.; Docquier, M.; Herrera, P.L.; Wilhelm, D.; et al. Insulin and IGF1 receptors are essential for XX and XY gonadal differentiation and adrenal development in mice. *PLoS Genet.* **2013**, *9*, e1003160. [CrossRef] [PubMed]
7. Cannarella, R.; Arato, I.; Condorelli, R.A.; Luca, G.; Barbagallo, F.; Alamo, A.; Bellucci, C.; Lilli, C.; La Vignera, S.; Calafiore, R.; et al. The IGF1 receptor is involved in follicle-stimulating hormone signaling in porcine neonatal sertoli cells. *J. Clin. Med.* **2019**, *8*, 577. [CrossRef] [PubMed]

8. Dupont, J.; Holzenberger, M. Biology of insulin-like growth factors in development. *Birth Defects Res. Part C Embryo Today* **2003**, *69*, 257–271. [CrossRef]
9. Nef, S.; Verma-Kurvari, S.; Merenmies, J.; Vassalli, J.D.; Efstratiadis, A.; Accili, D.; Parada, L.F. Testis determination requires insulin receptor family function in mice. *Nature* **2003**, *426*, 291–295. [CrossRef] [PubMed]
10. Pitetti, J.L.; Calvel, P.; Zimmermann, C.; Conne, B.; Papaioannou, M.D.; Aubry, F.; Cederroth, C.R.; Urner, F.; Fumel, B.; Crausaz, M.; et al. An essential role for insulin and IGF1 receptors in regulating sertoli cell proliferation, testis size, and FSH action in mice. *Mol. Endocrinol.* **2013**, *27*, 814–827. [CrossRef]
11. Levine, H.; Jørgensen, N.; Martino-Andrade, A.; Mendiola, J.; Weksler-Derri, D.; Mindlis, I.; Pinotti, R.; Swan, S.H. Temporal trends in sperm count: A systematic review and meta-regression analysis. *Hum. Reprod. Update* **2017**, *23*, 646–659. [CrossRef]
12. Finucane, M.M.; Stevens, G.A.; Cowan, M.J.; Danaei, G.; Lin, J.K.; Paciorek, C.J.; Singh, G.M.; Gutierrez, H.R.; Lu, Y.; Bahalim, A.N.; et al. Global burden of metabolic risk factors of chronic diseases collaborating group (body mass index). National, regional, and global trends in body-mass index since 1980: Systematic analysis of health examination surveys and epidemiological studies with 960 country-years and 9·1 million participants. *Lancet* **2011**, *377*, 557–567.
13. Winters, S.J.; Wang, C.; Abdelrahaman, E.; Hadeed, V.; Dyky, M.A.; Brufsky, A. Inhibin-B levels in healthy young adult men and prepubertal boys: Is obesity the cause for the contemporary decline in sperm count because of fewer Sertoli cells? *J. Androl.* **2006**, *27*, 560–564. [CrossRef] [PubMed]
14. Buyukinan, M.; Atar, M.; Pirgon, O.; Kurku, H.; Erdem, S.S.; Deniz, I. Anti-mullerian hormone and inhibin B levels in obese boys; Relations with cardiovascular risk factors. *Exp. Clin. Endocrinol. Diabetes* **2018**, *126*, 528–533. [CrossRef] [PubMed]
15. Hart, R.J.; Doherty, D.A.; Mori, T.A.; Adams, L.A.; Huang, R.C.; Minaee, N.; Handelsman, D.J.; McLachlan, R.; Norman, R.J.; Dickinson, J.E.; et al. Features of the metabolic syndrome in late adolescence are associated with impaired testicular function at 20 years of age. *Hum. Reprod.* **2019**, *34*, 389–402. [CrossRef] [PubMed]
16. Arato, I.; Luca, G.; Mancuso, F.; Bellucci, C.; Lilli, C.; Calvitti, M.; Hansen, B.C.; Milardi, D.; Grande, G.; Calafiore, R. An in vitro prototype of a porcine biomimetic testis-like cell culture system: A novel tool for the study of reassembled Sertoli and Leydig cells. *Asian J. Androl.* **2018**, *20*, 160–165. [PubMed]
17. Luca, G.; Mancuso, F.; Calvitti, M.; Arato, I.; Falabella, G.; Bufalari, A.; De Monte, V.; Tresoldi, E.; Nastruzzi, C.; Basta, G.; et al. Long-term stability, functional competence, and safety of microencapsulated specific pathogen-free neonatal porcine Sertoli cells: A potential product for cell transplant therapy. *Xenotransplantation* **2015**, *22*, 273–283. [CrossRef] [PubMed]
18. Mather, J.P.; Philip, D.D. Primary culture of testicular somatic cells. In *Methods for Serum Free Culture of Cells of the Endocrine System*; Barnes, D.W., Sirbasku, D.A., Sato, G.H., Eds.; Liss: New York, NY, USA, 1999; pp. 24–45.
19. Giovagnoli, S.; Mancuso, F.; Vannini, S.; Calvitti, M.; Piroddi, M.; Pietrella, D.; Arato, I.; Falabella, G.; Galli, F.; Moretti, M.; et al. Microparticle-loaded neonatal porcine Sertoli cells for cell-based therapeutic and drug delivery system. *J. Control. Release* **2014**, *192*, 249–261. [CrossRef]
20. Bradford, M.M. A rapid and sensitive method for the quantitation of microgram quantities of protein utilizing the principle of protein-dye binding. *Anal. Biochem.* **1976**, *72*, 248–254. [CrossRef]
21. Tasiou, V.; Hiber, M.; Steenpass, L. A mouse model for imprinting of the human retinoblastoma gene. *PLoS ONE* **2015**, *10*, e0134672. [CrossRef]
22. Li, B.; Berman, J.; Tang, J.T.; Lin, T.J. The early growth response factor-1 is involved in stem cell factor (SCF)-induced interleukin 13 production by mast cells, but is dispensable for SCF-dependent mast cell growth. *J. Biol. Chem.* **2007**, *282*, 22573–22581. [CrossRef] [PubMed]
23. Campbell, J.M.; Lane, M.; Owens, J.A.; Bakos, H.W. Paternal obesity negatively affects male fertility and assisted reproduction outcomes: A systematic review and meta-analysis. *Reprod. Biomed. Online* **2015**, *31*, 593–604. [CrossRef] [PubMed]
24. Ventimiglia, E.; Capogrosso, P.; Serino, A.; Boeri, L.; Colicchia, M.; La Croce, G.; Scano, R.; Papaleo, E.; Damiano, R.; Montorsi, F.; et al. Metabolic syndrome in White-European men presenting for secondary couple's infertility: An investigation of the clinical and reproductive burden. *Asian J. Androl.* **2017**, *19*, 368–373. [PubMed]

25. Condorelli, R.A.; La Vignera, S.; Mongioì, L.M.; Alamo, A.; Calogero, A.E. Diabetes mellitus and infertility: Different pathophysiological effects in type 1 and type 2 on sperm function. *Front. Endocrinol. (Lausanne)* **2018**, *9*, 268. [CrossRef] [PubMed]
26. Law, N.C.; Donaubauer, E.M.; Zeleznik, A.J.; Hunzicker-Dunn, M. How protein kinase A activates canonical tyrosine kinase signaling pathways to promote granulosa cell differentiation. *Endocrinology* **2017**, *17*, 2043–2051. [CrossRef] [PubMed]
27. Law, N.C.; Hunzicker-Dunn, M.E. Insulin receptor substrate 1, the hub linking follicle-stimulating hormone to phosphatidylinositol 3-kinase activation. *J. Biol. Chem.* **2016**, *291*, 4547–4560. [CrossRef] [PubMed]
28. Ren, L.; Zhou, X.; Huang, X.; Wang, C.; Li, Y. The IRS/PI3K/Akt signaling pathway mediates olanzapine-induced hepatic insulin resistance in male rats. *Life Sci.* **2019**, *217*, 229–236. [CrossRef]
29. Faure, M.; Guibert, E.; Alves, S.; Pain, B.; Ramé, C.; Dupont, J.; Brillard, J.P.; Froment, P. The insulin sensitiser metformin regulates chicken Sertoli and germ cell populations. *Reproduction* **2016**, *151*, 527–538. [CrossRef]
30. Rindone, G.M.; Gorga, A.; Regueira, M.; Pellizzari, E.H.; Cigorraga, S.B.; Galardo, M.N.; Meroni, S.B.; Riera, M.F. Metformin counteracts the effects of FSH on rat Sertoli cell proliferation. *Reproduction* **2018**, *156*, 93–101. [CrossRef]
31. Tartarin, P.; Moison, D.; Guibert, E.; Dupont, J.; Habert, R.; Rouiller-Fabre, V.; Frydman, N.; Pozzi, S.; Frydman, R.; Lecureuil, C.; et al. Metformin exposure affects human and mouse fetal testicular cells. *Hum. Reprod.* **2012**, *27*, 3304–3314. [CrossRef]

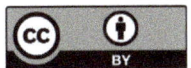

© 2019 by the authors. Licensee MDPI, Basel, Switzerland. This article is an open access article distributed under the terms and conditions of the Creative Commons Attribution (CC BY) license (http://creativecommons.org/licenses/by/4.0/).

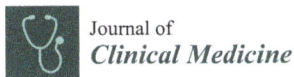 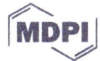

Article

The Risky Health Behaviours of Male Adolescents in the Southern Italian Region: Implications for Sexual and Reproductive Disease

Anna Perri [1,†], Danilo Lofaro [1,†], Giulia Izzo [2], Benedetta Aquino [1], Massimo Bitonti [3], Giuseppe Ciambrone [4], Sandro La Vignera [5], Carlotta Pozza [6], Daniele Gianfrilli [6] and Antonio Aversa [2,*]

1 Kidney and Transplantation Research Center, Department of Nephrology, Dialysis and Transplantation, Annunziata Hospital, 87100 Cosenza, Italy
2 Department of Experimental and Clinical Medicine, Magna Græcia University, 88100 Catanzaro, Italy
3 Procrea Private Practice Association, 88100 Catanzaro, Italy
4 AOU Materdomini, 88100 Catanzaro, Italy
5 Department of Clinical and Experimental Medicine, University of Catania, 95124 Catania, Italy
6 Department of Experimental Medicine, Sapienza University of Rome, 00185 Rome, Italy
* Correspondence: aversa@unicz.it; Tel.: +3909613647344
† The authors contributed equally to the paper.

Received: 5 July 2019; Accepted: 4 September 2019; Published: 8 September 2019

Abstract: Recent epidemiological studies suggest an increase of sexual and reproductive chronic diseases caused by problematic behaviours acquired during peri-pubertal age. The aims of our study were: (i) to investigate awareness of sexual transmitted infections (STIs) among adolescents; (ii) to describe the close relationship between possibly incorrect lifestyles during adolescence and reproductive and sexual disturbances during adulthood. The "Amico-Andrologo" survey is a permanent nationwide surveillance program supported by the Italian Ministry of Health. We administered a validated structured interview to investigate the lifestyle of adolescents and their knowledge of STIs. We selected a cohort of 360 male high-school students aged ≥18 years old. In this cohort, 150 (41.5%) were smokers while 59 (19.7%) smoked more than 10 cigarettes/day; 25 (9.3%) declared a consumption ≥6 drinks/weekend; and 65 (19.7%) were habitual cannabis consumers (at least twice/week). Among the sample of students selected, the main sources of sexual disease information were the internet and friends. The perceived level of knowledge on STIs was the same between students that used contraceptive methods and students that did not. The present results demonstrate that adolescents in Calabria do not receive appropriate information about risky health behaviours. Therefore, there is a necessity for specific educational programs to increase awareness of dangerous behaviours during the transitional age that is relevant for a safe sexual and reproductive adult life.

Keywords: adolescent; lifestyle; fertility; transitional age

1. Introduction

"Risky behaviours" are habits that may impact future well-being and are typical for adolescents [1,2]. The transition from childhood to adulthood is determined by a series of psycho-physical and hormonal changes. These changes are fundamental for the complete maturation of teenagers and for acceptance and respect by their peers [3]. It is well known that adolescence is crucial for the correct development and maturation of the genitourinary tract. Epidemiological data have demonstrated an increase in chronic sexual and reproductive diseases caused by risky behaviours developed during adolescence [4,5]. Alcohol and marijuana are the most common substances abused by adolescents [6]. On the one hand, ethanol interferes not only with the production of gonadal steroids by blocking GnRH cascade, but also increases the oxidative stress inducing damage of Leydig and Sertoli cell functions. This may lead to lower semen volume and sperm motility and morphological alterations [7]. On the other hand, cannabis, although it raises sexual desire, may hamper erectile function [8]. In fact, cannabis interferes with endothelial nitric oxide release, leading to vascular alterations in the absence of other risk factors [9]. In addition, the use of these substances often facilitates adolescents to have unprotected sexual intercourse with different partners, thus increasing their exposure to unwanted pregnancies and to Sexually Transmitted Infections (STIs) [10]. Studies on the sexual activity of Italian adolescents has shown that the age of one's first sexual intercourse is low (about 15.6 years old), and that 19.5% of new STI cases involve the youngest sexually active group (15–24 years old) [11,12]. STIs may contribute to male infertility, with Chlamydia trachomatis, Neisseria gonorrhoeae, and Herpes Papilloma Virus (HPV) infection being the most frequent pathogens in up to 15% of cases [13,14]. Even a heavy cigarette smoking habit may affect penile vasculature, reduce testosterone levels, and increase oxidative stress; therefore, cigarette use can influence semen volume and quality, leading to infertility [15].

In order to reduce the development of risky behaviours during adolescence, a series of health prevention and intervention campaigns have been conducted in the US. A first level approach was the Condom distribution program intended to prevent STIs [16]. A second, but no less important approach, was to encourage teens' communication with their extended family. Such relationships should be scheduled in teen health programs, which primarily focus on parents [17]. Although this latter aspect is considered a novel way to counteract risky behaviours among adolescents, it is not easily applied in specific social contexts.

Unfortunately, according to our knowledge, there are only a few adequate prevention programs aimed at changing sexual and reproductive attitudes among Italian teenagers, particularly in Southern Italian areas. The current study is a part of a nationwide andrological health surveillance program that was carried out on a sample of male adolescents attending their last year of High School in Calabria. The instrument of our survey was the administration of a questionnaire (an adaptation of the Centers for Disease Control and Prevention (CDC) Youth Risk Behaviours Surveillance (YRBS)) to estimate the prevalence of health risk behaviours.

2. Experimental Section

2.1. Subjects and Methods

The "Amico-Andrologo" Survey is a permanent national project conducted by the Italian Society of Andrology and Sexual Medicine (SIAMS) on young male adolescents attending the last year of high school, which was approved by the local Institutional Board Review, Regional School Authorities, and the Ministry of Health (protocol 19251/P—"Prevenzione in Andrologia" signed 28 April 2008). All male subjects were invited to complete an anonymous, self-administered, written questionnaire.

Between September 2016 and May 2017, we enrolled 360 male students (≥18 years old) attending high schools in the district of Cosenza, Catanzaro and Reggio di Calabria, Calabria area, Italy. The Survey investigated the adolescents' lifestyles (smoking habits, alcohol and drug consumption, and sexual behaviours and experiences) and explored the students' knowledge about STIs and major sources of information about these issues.

2.2. Statistical Analysis

All data are presented as the mean ± SD or count (%), as appropriate. A multiple comparison was performed using the Kruskal–Wallis test and Conover–Iman test for pairwise comparisons. The questionnaire data were collected and statistically elaborated by the R software (Version 3.5.3, The R Foundation for Statistical Computing).

3. Results

Health Risk Behaviors

The demographic characteristics of the participants are reported in Table 1. Since the adolescents interviewed were attending their last high-school year, they were all aged 18 or 19 (61.3% and 39.7%, respectively). Students enrolled were normal-weighted (BMI = 22.6 ± 3.1). According to their family situation, we discovered that 87 students (24.2%) had separated or divorced parents, and 14 (3.9%) had lost one or both of their parents. However, we found no association between demographic characteristics and substance abuse or problematic sexual habits.

Table 1. Clinical Features of enrolled students.

	Students (*n* = 360)
Age	
18	217 (61.3)
19	143 (39.7)
Weight (kg)	71.2 ± 10.6
High (cm)	177 ± 7.2
BMI (kg/m^2)	22.6 ± 3.1
Parental Divorce/Separation	87 (24.2)
Fatherless and/or motherless	14 (3.9)

The analysis of smoking habits revealed that, overall, 150 students (41.5%) reported smoking (Figure 1a). In more detail, 59 students (19.7%) reported smoking approximately 10 or more cigarettes/day (Figure 1b), and, surprisingly, 124 students (35.2%) smoked their first cigarette before 15 years of age (Table 2).

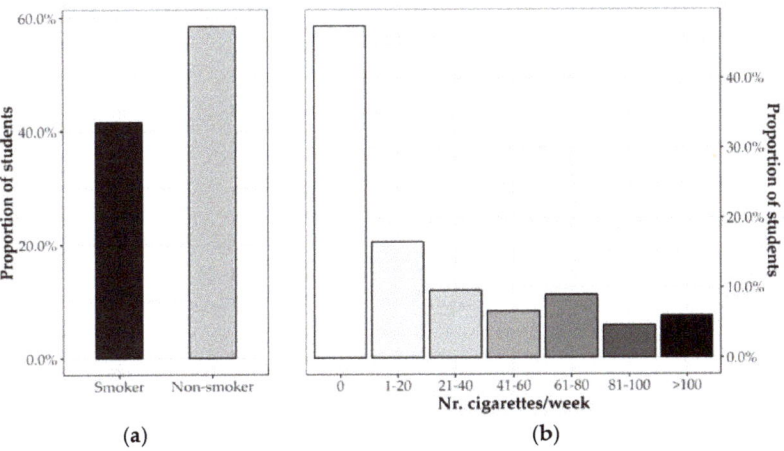

Figure 1. (**a**) Percent of smokers and non-smokers students and (**b**) number of cigarettes/day.

Table 2. Percentage of students divided by the different age of their first cigarette.

Age at First Cigarettes (%)	Students
never	114 (32.4)
≤8 (years)	5 (1.4)
9–10 (years)	12 (3.4)
11–12 (years)	36 (10.2)
13–14 (years)	71 (20.2)
15–16 (years)	85 (24.1)
≥17 (years)	29 (8.2)

According to alcohol consumption, only 25 students (9.3%) declared a consumption of ≥6 drinks per weekend (Figure 2).

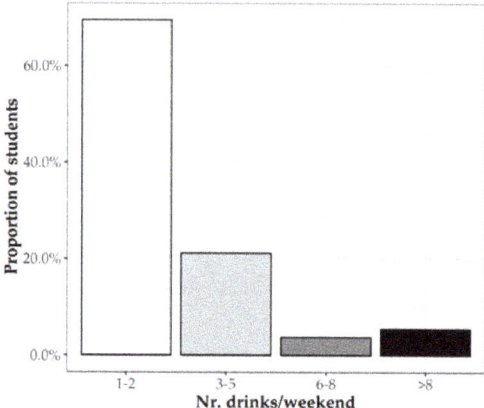

Figure 2. Number of alcoholic drinks/weekend.

For the consumption of illicit drugs, 65 students (19.7%) declared to be habitual cannabis smokers (at least twice a week; Figure 3a). Moreover, we found a linear association between cannabis and alcohol consumption ($p < 0.001$; Figure 3b).

Data on sexual education showed that the internet and peers were the main sources of information about sexuality, contraception, and STIs. On the other hand, only a few students stated that they had received sexual education from teachers, doctors, or relatives (Figure 4).

Interestingly, 242 (53.5%) of the 360 sexually active students examined admitted they use condoms; 65 students (25.6%) used contraceptive sometimes, while the remaining 53 (20.9%) declared they had never used them. Most of the students reported sufficient information about STIs: 61 students (17.7%) showed excellent knowledge, while 169 (49.0%) reported good knowledge. Surprisingly, these percentages were higher among those not using contraceptives at all (Figure 5).

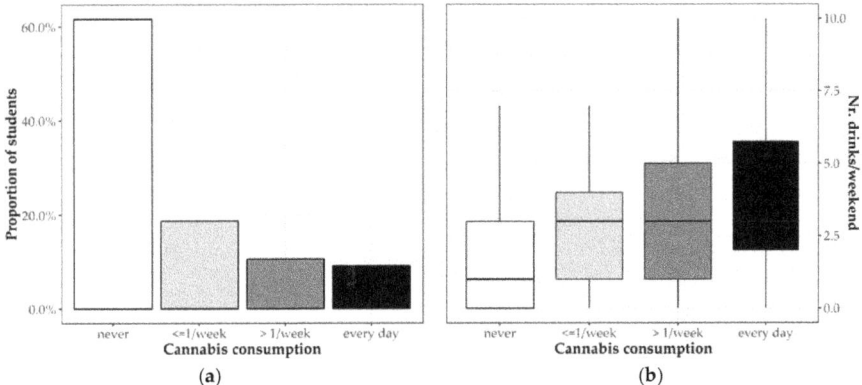

Figure 3. (a) Frequency of cannabis consumption among students and (b) the association between alcohol and cannabis consumption.

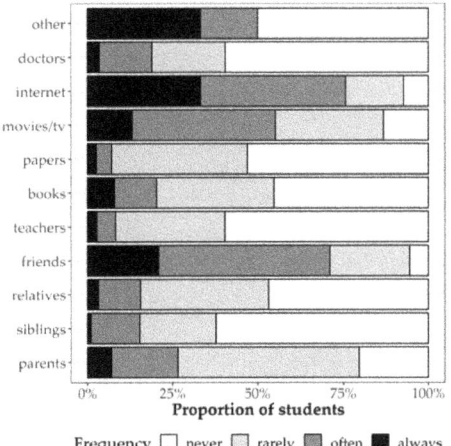

Figure 4. Percentage of the students' reported source for information on sexuality.

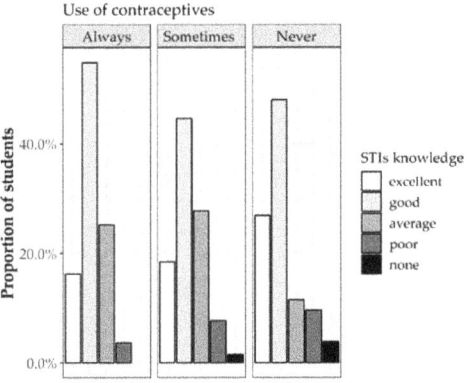

Figure 5. Perceived level of knowledge on STIs between students according to contraceptive use frequency.

4. Discussion

Our study is the first to show data on male adolescents' attitudes and risky behaviours in a Southern Italian region (Calabria). The results demonstrate that their consumption of cannabis and alcohol is lower compared to that of their peers living in Central or Northern Italian regions. Moreover, we found out that most of these adolescents receive information on sexuality and STIs mainly from the internet and friends and that a good knowledge of STIs was, surprisingly, associated with a habit to not use contraceptive methods.

It is well known that adolescence is associated with high levels of alcohol binge drinking because it encourages the initiation of sexual activity by lowering anxiety and inhibitions [18]. Unfortunately, chronic alcohol consumption is also associated with the appearance of sexual dysfunction, such as the loss of libido, premature ejaculation, and erectile dysfunction [19]. Adolescents also admit to the regular use of cannabis and other illicit drugs, risky behaviours that expose them to potential future sexual disturbances and diseases [20]. In addition, consumption of these substances is often continued throughout their adult lives, with further negative consequences on sexuality and fertility [9].

In contrast with our results, Gianfrilli et al. have recently reported that in several Northern and Central Italian regions, just one over half (51%) of the subjects examined admitted to being regular cigarette smokers. Even the percentages related to occasional alcohol consumption (80%) and heavy drinking habits (30%) were much higher when compared to the results of our study [21]. One point in common with Gianfrilli's study is that adolescents try illegal drugs, especially marijuana/hashish, at an early age. Cigarette smokers are also equally represented in all Italian regions. The consumption of alcohol (per weekend = 9.3%) and cannabis (least once-a-week = 21%) were lower in Southern regions than in Northern ones. Interestingly, we observed that the use of alcohol and cannabis among adolescents in Southern regions is often combined. This finding had already been reported by other authors in a survey conducted on young people ages 13 to 19 [22].

Luckily, recent studies have demonstrated that, since the early 2000s, the consumption of tobacco, alcohol, and cannabis among adolescents is decreasing both in Europe and North America [23,24]. In fact, the International Health Behaviour in School-aged Children (HBSC) study showed that the percentage of 15 year old smokers in Europe and North America decreased from 24% in 2002 to 12% in 2014. Weekly alcohol consumption decreased from 29% to 13%, and, finally, the habit of cannabis smoking among 15 year old boys decreased from 22% to 15% [25,26]. These changes may be due to a sharp drop in face-to-face peer contacts that yielded an increased use of electronic media communications [27]. The results of the studies conducted in Northern, Central, and Southern Italian regions are in contrast with these findings and, therefore, suggest that Italian adolescents need more information and awareness about the dangers of risky behaviours. Thus, it is advisable to promote a series of robust campaigns in Italian regions aimed at changing the attitudes of adolescents regarding the excessive use of tobacco/marijuana.

Gianfrilli et al. showed that 60.3% of adolescents engage in regular sexual activity and, among them, 41% have unprotected sex [21]. Our results highlight a discrepancy between the belief that adolescents have good knowledge of the risks related to unprotected sex and their habit not to use condoms, even with different partners. Indeed, although about 70% of the respondents declared to know about STIs, we observed that 25.6% of students examined used contraceptive "sometimes" and that the 20.9% of them used contraceptives "never". These findings are in line with reported data in the literature. The survey conducted by Drago et al. on 2867 Italian adolescents, which aimed to investigate knowledge about sexuality, revealed that 22% of the interviewees knew that condoms are the only contraceptive means for preventing STIs, and just 0.5% have recognized sexual diseases on the list provided [11]. Similar results have been reported by Bergamini et al, whose study pointed out the need to improve teenagers' awareness of risky behaviours for the prevention of STIs. In their opinion, school should play a crucial role in the reinforcement of sexual educational programs [28]. The survey of Wand et al., carried out on a sample of 16–29 year old subjects, demonstrated that the majority of high risk sexual behaviours and STI diagnoses were associated with the consumption of illicit drugs and alcohol. In conclusion, the diffusion of STIs could be prevented by mitigating high risky sexual behaviours among teenagers [29].

As we have already stated before, another risky behaviour among adolescents is represented by their attitude to have unprotected sexual intercourse. This dangerous habit predisposes male adolescents to the development of male accessory gland infections (MAGI), including prostatitis, vesiculitis, and/or epididymitis. Several kinds of microorganisms are involved in the etiology of MAGI, such as *Escherichia coli*, *Neisseria gonorrhoeae*, *Chlamydia trachomatis*, *Ureaplasma urealyticum*, *Mycoplasma hominis*, and other mycoplasmas, *Candida albicans*, *Trichomonas vaginalis*, and HPV [30]. We believe that a good information campaign is necessary both for families and adolescents, to contrast problematic habits in sexual intercourse. It is also advisable that HPV vaccination in 11 year old boys become mandatory in order to prevent the spread of STIs and other diseases not directly related to HPV. This new practice would likely contribute to a sharp reduction in the chronic, often asymptomatic, damage responsible for apparently idiopathic sperm abnormalities. Asymptomatic or pauci-symptomatic forms can lead to chronic inflammatory processes, responsible for the development of hypertrophic-congestive and fibro-sclerotic ultrasound-evidenced variants. These forms differently impact sperm quality, sometimes irreversibly [19]. They also may contribute to sexual dysfunction, such premature ejaculation [31].

In general, although the attitudes and sexual behaviours of the population have radically changed, adolescents usually approach sexuality unprepared and uninformed, especially when they live in underdeveloped socio-economic and cultural contexts. In addition, as we have already discussed, a high percentage of teenagers learn about these issues on the internet and compare what they know with their friends [32]. Unfortunately, the internet is just a container of general (and sometimes incorrect) information, ranging from pornography to (un)controlled medical indications that cannot provide the web-surfer with adequate interpretative tools. Several studies have shown that interpersonal relationships are the primary elements in the decision-making of adolescents in risky sexual behaviours and that peers are more important than adults in defining norms and attitudes [10,33].

We are aware that the limitations of the present study are related to the lack of data on testicular volume, sperm parameters and sexual function. We also recognize that a multicenter prospective study should be carried out to assess the impact of risky health behaviours on sexuality and fertility per year of exposure, starting from adolescence. However, we have to point out that this study, which is unique and relevant because of the novelty of its results, represents a different approach compared to previous epidemiological data coming from prevention campaigns in Calabrian areas.

5. Conclusions

Data from the present survey suggest that in Calabria, risky health behaviours are wide spread among male teenagers. Adolescents still do not acquire appropriate education about sexual and reproductive health behaviours because of their unreliable sources of information—peers or the internet, instead of institutional figures. Another negative attitude that affects adolescents' sexual and reproductive lives is represented by their high alcohol and cannabis consumption during the convivial weekend meetings.

Therefore, it is necessary to promote focused educational programs, starting post-puberty, in order to make families and teenagers aware of the impact of MAGI on male fertility and sexuality.

We also recommend sensitizing young boys to the use of condoms, to mitigate the high spread of HPV and other STIs. Regarding this aspect, HPV vaccination in 11 year old boys could represent a fundamental element for the primary prevention of STIs, and even of other diseases not directly related to HPV.

In conclusion, we suggest involving families and schoolteachers in future information campaigns addressed to teenagers. A correct institutional information campaign is, in fact, the only way to produce a safe sexual and reproductive life in adulthood.

Author Contributions: Conceptualization of the study: A.A., D.G., and A.P.; methodology, software, formal analysis and data curation: D.L.; validation: G.I., B.A., S.L.V., C.P., M.B., and G.C.; investigation: G.I.; writing—original draft preparation: A.P. and D.L.; writing—review and editing: A.A.; visualization: D.G.; supervision: S.L.V. and D.G.; Project administration: A.A. and D.G.

Funding: This research was funded by the National Centre for Disease Prevention and Control of the Italian Ministry of Health as part of the 'Prevention in Andrology' project (protocol 19251/P—'Prevenzione in Andrologia' signed 28 April 2008). None of the authors received any forms of compensation by pharmaceutical companies or agencies for their work in this project. The authors had full access to all data in the study and share full responsibility for the decision to submit this article for publication.

Acknowledgments: We thank Maria Regolo for the English revision of the manuscript.

Conflicts of Interest: Nothing to discard. The authors declare that funders had no role in the design of the study, in the collection, analyses, or interpretation of data, in the writing of the manuscript, or in the decision to publish the results.

References

1. Kwan, M.Y.; Cairney, J.; Faulkner, G.E.; Pullenayegum, E.E. Physical activity and other health-risk behaviors during the transition into early adulthood: A longitudinal cohort study. *Am. J. Prev. Med.* **2012**, *42*, 14–20. [CrossRef] [PubMed]
2. Pampel, F.C.; Mollborn, S.; Lawrence, E.M. Life course transitions in early adulthood and SES disparities in tobacco use. *Soc. Sci. Res.* **2014**, *43*, 45–59. [CrossRef] [PubMed]
3. Jessor, R. Problem Behavior Theory and Adolescent Risk Behavior: A Re-Formulation. In *The Origins and Development of Problem Behavior Theory: The Collected Works of Richard Jessor*; Jessor, R., Ed.; Springer International Publishing: Cham, Switzerland, 2016; pp. 117–130.
4. Abreu, A.P.; Kaiser, U.B. Pubertal development and regulation. *Lancet Diabetes Endocrinol.* **2016**, *4*, 254–264. [CrossRef]
5. Sansone, A.; Di Dato, C.; de Angelis, C.; Menafra, D.; Pozza, C.; Pivonello, R.; Isidori, A.; Gianfrilli, D. Smoke, alcohol and drug addiction and male fertility. *Reprod. Biol. Endocrinol.* **2018**, *16*, 3. [CrossRef] [PubMed]
6. Gillman, A.S.; Yeater, E.A.; Feldstein Ewing, S.W.; Kong, A.S.; Bryan, A.D. Risky Sex in High-Risk Adolescents: Associations with Alcohol Use, Marijuana Use, and Co-Occurring Use. *AIDS Behav.* **2018**, *22*, 1352–1362. [CrossRef] [PubMed]
7. Durairajanayagam, D. Lifestyle causes of male infertility. *Arab J. Urol.* **2018**, *16*, 10–20. [CrossRef]
8. Shamloul, R.; Bella, A.J. Impact of cannabis use on male sexual health. *J. Sex. Med.* **2011**, *8*, 971–975. [CrossRef] [PubMed]
9. Aversa, A.; Rossi, F.; Francomano, D.; Bruzziches, R.; Bertone, C.; Santiemma, V.; Spera, G. Early endothelial dysfunction as a marker of vasculogenic erectile dysfunction in young habitual cannabis users. *Int. J. Impot. Res.* **2008**, *20*, 566–573. [CrossRef]
10. Widman, L.; Choukas-Bradley, S.; Helms, S.W.; Prinstein, M.J. Adolescent Susceptibility to Peer Influence in Sexual Situations. *J. Adolesc. Health* **2016**, *58*, 323–329. [CrossRef]
11. Drago, F.; Ciccarese, G.; Zangrillo, F.; Gasparini, G.; Cogorno, L.; Riva, S.; Javor, S.; Cozzani, E.; Broccolo, F.; Esposito, S.; et al. A Survey of Current Knowledge on Sexually Transmitted Diseases and Sexual Behaviour in Italian Adolescents. *Int. J. Environ. Res. Public Health* **2016**, *13*, 422. [CrossRef]
12. Panatto, D.; Amicizia, D.; Lugarini, J.; Sasso, T.; Sormani, M.P.; Badolati, G.; Gasparini, R. Sexual behaviour in Ligurian (Northern Italy) adolescents and young people: Suggestions for HPV vaccination policies. *Vaccine* **2009**, *27* (Suppl. 1), A6–A10. [CrossRef]
13. Akgul, A.; Kadioglu, A.; Koksal, M.O.; Ozmez, A.; Agacfidan, A. Sexually transmitted agents and their association with leucocytospermia in infertility clinic patients. *Andrologia* **2018**, *50*, e13127. [CrossRef] [PubMed]

14. Lyu, Z.; Feng, X.; Li, N.; Zhao, W.; Wei, L.; Chen, Y.; Yang, W.; Ma, H.; Yao, B.; Zhang, K.; et al. Human papillomavirus in semen and the risk for male infertility: A systematic review and meta-analysis. *BMC Infect. Dis.* **2017**, *17*, 714. [CrossRef] [PubMed]
15. Ilacqua, A.; Izzo, G.; Emerenziani, G.P.; Baldari, C.; Aversa, A. Lifestyle and fertility: The influence of stress and quality of life on male fertility. *Reprod. Biol. Endocrinol.* **2018**, *16*, 115. [CrossRef] [PubMed]
16. McCool-Myers, M. Implementing condom distribution programs in the United States: Qualitative insights from program planners. *Eval. Program. Plan.* **2019**, *74*, 20–26. [CrossRef] [PubMed]
17. Grossman, J.M.; Lynch, A.D.; Richer, A.M.; De Souza, L.M.; Ceder, I. Extended-Family Talk about Sex and Teen Sexual Behavior. *Int. J. Environ. Res. Public Health* **2019**, *6*, 480. [CrossRef] [PubMed]
18. Prabhakaran, D.K.; Nisha, A.; Varghese, P.J. Prevalence and correlates of sexual dysfunction in male patients with alcohol dependence syndrome: A cross-sectional study. *Indian J. Psychiatry* **2018**, *60*, 71–77. [CrossRef]
19. La Vignera, S.; Vicari, E.; Condorelli, R.; D'Agata, R.; Calogero, A.E. Hypertrophic-congestive and fibro-sclerotic ultrasound variants of male accessory gland infection have different sperm output. *J. Endocrinol. Investig.* **2011**, *34*, e330–e335. [CrossRef]
20. Ross, J.M.; Granja, K.; Duperrouzel, J.C.; Pacheco-Colon, I. Risky sexual behavior among adolescents: The role of decision-making, problems from cannabis use and externalizing disorder symptoms. *J. Clin. Exp. Neuropsychol.* **2019**, *41*, 300–311. [CrossRef]
21. Gianfrilli, D.; Ferlin, A.; Isidori, A.M.; Garolla, A.; Maggi, M.; Pivonello, R.; Santi, D.; Sansone, A.; Balercia, G.; Granata, A.R.M.; et al. Risk behaviours and alcohol in adolescence are negatively associated with testicular volume: Results from the Amico-Andrologo survey. *Andrology* **2019**. [CrossRef]
22. Chivandire, C.T.; January, J. Correlates of cannabis use among high school students in Shamva District, Zimbabwe: A descriptive cross-sectional study. *Malawi Med. J.* **2016**, *28*, 53–56. [CrossRef] [PubMed]
23. De Looze, M.; Ter Bogt, T.F.; Raaijmakers, Q.A.; Pickett, W.; Kuntsche, E.; Vollebergh, W.A. Cross-national evidence for the clustering and psychosocial correlates of adolescent risk behaviours in 27 countries. *Eur. J. Public Health* **2015**, *25*, 50–56. [CrossRef] [PubMed]
24. Hublet, A.; Bendtsen, P.; de Looze, M.E.; Fotiou, A.; Donnelly, P.; Vilhjalmsson, R.; Baska, T.; Aasvee, K.; Franelic, I.P.; Nic Gabhainn, S.; et al. Trends in the co-occurrence of tobacco and cannabis use in 15-year-olds from 2002 to 2010 in 28 countries of Europe and North America. *Eur. Public Health* **2015**, *25* (Suppl. 2), 73–75. [CrossRef]
25. Currie, C.; Roberts, C.; Settertobulte, W.; Morgan, A.; Smith, R.; Samdal, O.; World Health Organization. *Young People's Health in Context: Health Behaviour in School-Aged Children (HBSC) Study: International Report from the 2001/2002 Survey*; World Health Organization Regional Office for Europe: Geneva, Switzerland, 2004.
26. Inchley, J.; Currie, D.B.; Young, T.; Samdal, O.; Torsheim, T.; Augustson, L.; Mathison, F.; Aleman-Diaz, A.Y.; Molcho, M.; World Health Organization. *Growing up Unequal: Gender and Socioeconomic Differences in Young People's Health and Well-Being: Health Behaviour in School-Aged Children (HBSC) Study: International Report from the 2013/2014 Survey*; World Health Organization Regional Office for Europe: Geneva, Switzerland, 2016.
27. De Looze, M.; van Dorsselaer, S.; Stevens, G.; Boniel-Nissim, M.; Vieno, A.; Van den Eijnden, R. The decline in adolescent substance use across Europe and North America in the early twenty-first century: A result of the digital revolution? *Int. J. Public Health* **2019**, *64*, 229–240. [CrossRef] [PubMed]
28. Bergamini, M.; Cucchi, A.; Guidi, E.; Stefanati, A.; Bonato, B.; Lupi, S.; Gregorio, P. Risk perception of sexually transmitted diseases and teenage sexual behaviour: Attitudes towards in a sample of Italian adolescents. *J. Prev. Med. Hyg.* **2013**, *54*, 114–119. [PubMed]
29. Wand, H.; Ward, J.; Bryant, J.; Delaney-Thiele, D.; Worth, H.; Pitts, M.; Kaldor, J.M. Individual and population level impacts of illicit drug use, sexual risk behaviours on sexually transmitted infections among young Aboriginal and Torres Strait Islander people: Results from the GOANNA survey. *BMC Public Health* **2016**, *16*, 600. [CrossRef]
30. La Vignera, S.; Vicari, E.; Condorelli, R.A.; Franchina, C.; Scalia, G.; Morgia, G.; Perino, A.; Schillaci, R.; Calogero, A.E. Prevalence of human papilloma virus infection in patients with male accessory gland infection. *Reprod. Biomed. Online* **2015**, *30*, 385–391. [CrossRef]
31. La Vignera, S.; Condorelli, R.A.; Vicari, E.; Favilla, V.; Morgia, G.; Calogero, A.E. Acquired premature ejaculation and male accessory gland infection: Relevance of ultrasound examination. *Asian J. Androl.* **2016**, *18*, 769–772. [CrossRef]

32. Zani, B. L'adolescente e la sessualità. In *Psicologia Dell'adolescenza*; Zani, B., Ed.; IL Mulino: Bologna, Italy, 1997; pp. 189–208.
33. Pombeni, M.L. L'adolescente e i gruppi di coetanei. In *Psicologia Dell'adolescenza*; Pombeni, M.L., Ed.; IL Mulino: Bologna, Italy, 1993; pp. 225–244.

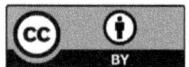
© 2019 by the authors. Licensee MDPI, Basel, Switzerland. This article is an open access article distributed under the terms and conditions of the Creative Commons Attribution (CC BY) license (http://creativecommons.org/licenses/by/4.0/).

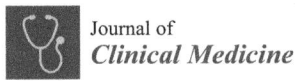 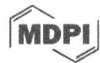

Review
Substance Abuse and Male Hypogonadism

Ylenia Duca [1], Antonio Aversa [2], Rosita Angela Condorelli [1], Aldo Eugenio Calogero [1] and Sandro La Vignera [1,*]

[1] Department of Clinical and Experimental Medicine, University of Catania, 95123 Catania, Italy; ylenia.duca@gmail.com (Y.D.); rosita.condorelli@unict.it (R.A.C.); acaloger@unict.it (A.E.C.)
[2] Department of Experimental and Clinical Medicine, University Magna Graecia of Catanzaro, 88100 Catanzaro, Italy; aversa@unicz.it
* Correspondence: sandrolavignera@unict.it

Received: 1 May 2019; Accepted: 18 May 2019; Published: 22 May 2019

Abstract: Progressive deterioration of male reproductive function is occurring in Western countries. Environmental factors and unhealthy lifestyles have been implicated in the decline of testosterone levels and sperm production observed in the last fifty years. Among unhealthy lifestyles, substance and drug abuse is a recognized cause of possible alterations of steroidogenesis and spermatogenesis. Alcohol, opioids and anabolic-androgenic steroids are capable to reduce testosterone production in male interfering with testicular and/or hypothalamic-pituitary function. Other substances such as nicotine, cannabis, and amphetamines alter spermatogenesis inducing oxidative stress and subsequent apoptosis in testicular tissue. Substance and drug abuse is a potentially reversible cause of hypogonadism, defined as the failure of the testis to produce physiological concentrations of testosterone and/or a normal number of spermatozoa. The identification of the abuse is important because the withdrawal of substance intake can reverse the clinical syndrome. This review summarizes the most important clinical and experimental evidence on the effect of substance abuse on testosterone and sperm production.

Keywords: hypogonadism; oligozoospermia; substance abuse; drug abuse; alcohol; cigarette smoking; cannabis; amphetamines; opioids; anabolic-androgenic steroids

---

1. Introduction

According to the most recent definition, hypogonadism is a clinical syndrome resulting from the failure of the testis to produce physiological concentrations of testosterone and/or a normal number of spermatozoa due to pathologies of the hypothalamic–pituitary–testicular axis [1].

Pathogenic noxae acting at testicular level give rise to a syndrome characterized by low testosterone concentrations, impairment of spermatogenesis, and elevated gonadotropin levels, defined as primary hypogonadism. Otherwise, secondary hypogonadism is caused by a dysfunction of the hypothalamus–pituitary unit, resulting in low testosterone concentrations, impairment of spermatogenesis, and low or inappropriately normal gonadotropin levels [1]. Hypogonadism is defined as organic when a congenital, structural, or destructive disorder results in a permanent dysfunction, and functional when potentially reversible conditions suppress temporarily gonadotropin and/or testosterone production [1].

The diagnosis of hypogonadism can be formulated when at least two testosterone values below normal are found in patients with symptoms and signs of testosterone deficiency. Testosterone must be measured in morning samples after a fast of at least 8 hours. To uniform reference values among laboratories and assays, the Endocrine Society recently proposed a harmonized reference range, according to which total testosterone values should be considered reduced if lower than 264 ng/dL or 9.2 nmol/L [1]. The measurement of free testosterone is not routinely recommended; however, it can be useful in patients with altered sex hormone-binding globulin (SHBG) concentrations. Indeed, only 2–4% of testosterone circulates in free form, while the remainder is bound to SHBG and, less tenaciously, to albumin. In conditions when SHGB levels are reduced (e.g., obesity, type 2 diabetes mellitus, androgen use), total testosterone concentrations could be below normal values even if free testosterone levels are in the normal range. The gold standard for free testosterone measurement is the equilibrium dialysis method. However, most laboratories use immunoassays that are less accurate. In this case, to calculate free testosterone starting from total testosterone, SHBG, and albumin values is preferable [1].

Symptoms and signs suggestive of testosterone deficiency include reduced libido and sexual activity, decreased spontaneous erections, erectile dysfunction, gynecomastia, infertility, osteopenia/osteoporosis, hot flushes, and sweats. Other non-specific symptoms, such as fatigue, depressed mood, poor concentration and memory, sleep disturbance, reduced muscle mass and strength, increased body fat and body mass index [1], although not decisive for defining the diagnosis, are important from a clinical point of view because they have a great impact on the quality of life of hypogonadal patients.

The prevalence of hypogonadism is rising over time, not only for the improvement in diagnostic procedures. In 2007, Travison and colleagues analyzed data from the Massachusetts Male Aging Study (MMAS) about testosterone concentration and observed an overtime decline in total testosterone levels higher than that attributable to aging. The Author hypothesized that the recorded age-independent population decrease in testosterone could be attributable to birth cohort differences or to environmental factors [2]. The same trend has been shown in Europe. Data from Danish population surveys conducted from 1982 to 2001 evidenced a secular trend in testosterone and SHBG serum levels among age-matched men, with lower levels in the younger men and in those more recently studied [3].

The progressive deterioration of male reproductive function also affects sperm production. In 2017, Levine and colleagues performed a systematic review and meta-regression analysis, showing that sperm concentration in Western countries declined by 1.4% per year, with an overall decline of 52.4%, between 1973 and 2011. Similarly, total sperm count in the same period declined by 1.6% per year, with an overall decline of 59.3%. No trend in concentration and total sperm count reduction was found in other countries [4].

Factors that could contribute to the worsening of testicular function in Western countries include the progressive increase in visceral adiposity among the population, changes in lifestyle and behaviors, environmental pollution and exposure to endocrine-disrupting compounds (i.e., phthalates) [5]. Among unhealthy behaviors, alcohol abuse, cigarette smoking, excessive caffeine intake, illicit drug intake, opioid consumption, and inappropriate use of anabolic steroids have been studied as a possible cause of reduced sperm production and/or reduced testosterone levels in hypogonadal men [6].

In our review, we summarized the most important clinical and experimental evidence on the effect of substance abuse on testosterone and sperm production For many of the substances examined most of the evidence comes from in vivo and in vitro animal studies or from retrospective human studies. Indeed, for ethical reasons, no intervention studies on humans can be performed. Unfortunately, data obtained in animals are not always reproducible in humans; so some aspects regarding the mechanisms of action of several substances on the reproductive function must be further clarified.

2. Alcohol

Since ancient times the consumption of alcoholic beverages has been part of the socio-cultural heritage of most populations. However, chronic and acute alcohol abuse is involved in the pathogenesis of many diseases, including liver diseases, cancers, cardiovascular disease, and neuropsychiatric disorders. The effects of alcohol intake on male reproductive function have also been evaluated, in vitro and in vivo. Both testosterone production and spermatogenesis seem to be affected by alcohol abuse in a dose-dependent manner: heavy drinkers are more likely to have a poor testicular function than moderate consumers.

2.1. Effects on Testosterone Production

It has been demonstrated that alcohol could decrease testosterone blood concentration acting both on testicular and central (hypothalamic and pituitary) level [7].

Since the 1980s, it is known that ethanol and acetaldehyde are important Leydig cells toxins. Van Thiel and colleagues performed both in vivo and in vitro studies assessing the alcohol effect on Leydig cells function [8]. In their in vivo human study, they evaluated the hormonal status of chronic alcoholic men, comparing it with that of healthy volunteers to whom a quantity of ethanol corresponding to a pint of whiskey/day was given for 30 days. They showed that almost all alcoholic men had low-normal or low testosterone levels and increased gonadotropin levels. In the healthy male volunteers, testosterone levels began to reduce from the baseline after 72 hours of ethanol ingestion and reached levels similar than those of alcoholic men after 30 days, while gonadotropins remained in the normal range [8]. In their in vivo animal studies, they showed that alcohol-fed rats had testosterone levels reduced by half compared to isocaloric non-alcohol fed rats [8]. In in vitro studies, they showed that rat testes perfused with ethanol and acetaldehyde showed a reduced production and secretion of testosterone in a dose-dependent manner. The same phenomenon occurred in cultured rat Leydig cells [8].

The reduced production of testosterone by Leydig cells is due to the inhibitory action of alcohol on the enzymes 3β-hydroxysteroid dehydrogenase and 17-ketosteroid reductase, which catalyze respectively the conversion from pregnenolone to progesterone and from androstenedione to testosterone. Progesterone is the precursor for the synthesis of testosterone, so its lack could lead to a decreased production of testosterone [9]. Furthermore, alcohol enhances the production of radical oxygen species that suppress the expression of the steroidogenic acute regulatory protein (StAR), which regulates the rate-limiting step in the steroid hormone biosynthesis that is the transport of cholesterol from the outer to inner mitochondrial membrane [10].

The decreased testosterone concentration in heavy drinkers depends on the reduced production by Leydig cells but also on the increased metabolism of androgens. It has been demonstrated that alcohol induces the enzyme aromatase that catalyzes the conversion of testosterone in estradiol and androstenedione in estrone [11].

The degree of testicular failure in alcoholic men seems to be related also to the extent of liver damage. A study evaluated testosterone and estradiol levels in patients subdivided into three groups according to the histological severity of liver damage: fatty change, hepatitis, and cirrhosis. Median estradiol levels were above the normal range in males of all three histological categories. Median testosterone concentrations were below the normal range in men with hepatitis and cirrhosis but not in those with fatty liver. Testosterone/SHBG ratio was reduced in patients with cirrhosis. Furthermore, estradiol and testosterone concentrations showed a negative correlation with serum albumin [12].

Although chronic alcohol abuse causes hypogonadism mainly through testicular damage, as evidenced by the high levels of gonadotropins found in most alcoholic men, alcohol is also able to act on the hypothalamus-pituitary axis and its effects at central level are more evident during acute ingestion. Ida and colleagues studied the effect of acute and repeated alcohol administration on plasma prolactin, luteinizing hormone (LH) and testosterone on adult healthy male volunteers [13]. They found that prolactin increased and testosterone decreased after thirty minutes from acute alcohol ingestion, but returned quite rapidly at baseline levels, while LH levels did not change significantly. The repeated alcohol ingestion over seven consecutive evenings did not lead to the development of tolerance to these hormonal changes. The Author hypothesized that alcohol might inhibit the release of hypothalamic dopamine to the hypophyseal-portal system and that hyperprolactinemia could be partially responsible for testosterone decrease after acute alcohol assumption [13]. Otherwise, in chronic abuse, alcohol seems not to affect prolactin levels [9].

A direct action of alcohol at pituitary level, resulting in the inhibition of LH release, has also been hypothesized. In animal models, the suppression of β-LH gene expression and protein release from the pituitary gland after ethanol exposure has been demonstrated [14]. Furthermore, alcohol is able to increase dose-dependently β-endorphin-like peptides release from the hypothalamus. β-endorphin can, in turn, suppress the production and release of gonadotropin-releasing hormone (GnRH) at neuronal level, and of testosterone from the testis [15]. Finally, the high estrogen levels found in alcoholic men can exert negative feedback on gonadotropin release contributing to further reduce testosterone production with a central mechanism [14].

The increase in estrogens concentration due to the enhanced testosterone and androstenedione aromatization and to the altered estrogens' breakdown by the damaged liver, together with the reduction in testosterone production, is responsible for the gynecomastia that frequently occurs in alcoholic cirrhotic patients [14].

2.2. Effects on Spermatogenesis

In the 1980s, Van Thiel and colleagues obtained testicular histology from five chronic alcoholic men and observed a profile characterized by loss of germ cells, peritubular fibrosis and collapse, and aggregate of residual Leydig cells between the abnormal seminiferous tubules [8]. They found the same histologic profile in alcohol-fed rats [8].

Ten years later, prospective autopsy studies showed that spermatogenic arrest and Sertoli cells-only syndrome are present in, respectively, 50% and 10% of heavy drinkers, while less than 20% of non-alcoholic controls have alterations of spermatogenesis [16]. The testicular damage was not related to the extent of liver damage because most of the men with Sertoli cells-only syndrome had not cirrhosis, but it was strongly correlated with daily alcohol intake: testicular alterations were more likely to be present in men who drank more than 80 g of alcohol daily [17].

More recent studies demonstrated that the reduction of testicular germ cells in alcoholic men is due to the activation of apoptosis. In the mouse testis, ethanol-induced apoptosis through the increased expression of Fas/Fas-L and p53, the up-regulation of Bax/Bcl-2 ratio, and the activation of caspase-3 [10].

The testicular histological alterations found in heavy drinkers clinically translate in a significant reduction in sperm, up to azoospermia [9]. The spermatogenetic damage caused by alcohol abuse seems to be reversible. Case reports and animal studies showed that spontaneous recovery of spermatogenesis could occur starting from 10–12 weeks after alcohol consumption withdrawal [18–21].

Unlike alcohol abuse, a moderate alcohol intake seems not associated with altered sperm concentration [22]. A dose-dependent effect was demonstrated by Jensen and colleagues, who found a progressive deterioration of sperm count, concentration and morphology with the increase in the amount of alcohol consumed, more evident in patients with a weekly alcohol intake higher than 25 units [23]. This trend has been recently confirmed: Boeri and colleagues showed that heavy drinking was associated with a lower sperm concentration than moderate drinking and/or abstaining. They also reported that drinking and smoking concomitantly has an even greater detrimental effect on semen parameters [24]. A recent meta-analysis assessed the association between alcohol intake and semen quality, examining the pooled data of fifteen cross-sectional studies, with a total of 16,395 enrolled men. Results showed a detrimental effect of alcohol on semen volume and sperm morphology but not on sperm concentration [25]. However, most of the studies included in the analysis evaluated men with moderate alcohol intake or did not report the exact alcohol intake of the patients. Anyway, results confirm that occasional alcohol consumption did not adversely affect semen parameters [25]. Some evidence indicate even a positive effect of moderate alcohol intake on semen quality [26].

It has been demonstrated that the homozygous deletion of the glutathione S-transferase (GST)-M1 gene increases the susceptibility to develop alcoholic liver cirrhosis in response to the toxic effects of alcohol chronic abuse [27]. Similarly, the association between alcohol-induced alteration of human spermatogenesis and GST-M1 genotype has been investigated. An autopsy study revealed that heavy drinkers with GST-M1 'null' genotype developed less frequently disorders of spermatogenesis; so, Authors hypothesized the GST M1 locus may be associated with susceptibility to alcohol-induced testicular damage [28].

A state of protein malnutrition, with nutritional imbalance or deficiencies, could contribute to the onset of spermatogenesis disorders, as well as testosterone deficiency, in alcoholic men. Due to low dietary intake or excessive loss (i.e., by vomiting or diarrhea), alcoholic patients can suffer from the lack of some minerals and micronutrients such as zinc, magnesium, folate, and vitamins (A, D, E), belonging to the human not enzymatic antioxidant system. The lowering of antioxidant defenses exposes the germ cells to the deleterious effect of oxidative stress [29].

3. Cigarette Smoking

Even more than alcohol, cigarette smoking is recognized as a risk factor for many diseases: cardiovascular diseases, lung diseases, malignant neoplasms, etc. Since the 1980s, scientific literature has been interested in evaluating the effects of cigarette smoking on reproductive function. Tobacco smoke is a complex mixture of over than 8,700 substances. Harmful cigarette smoke constituents include carbon monoxide, nitrogen oxide, ammonia, heavy metals, various polycyclic aromatic hydrocarbons and aldehydes, such as hydroquinone, catechol, acrolein, crotonaldehyde, and formaldehyde [30]. Recently, even nicotine, the major psychoactive substance in cigarette smoke, has been called into question in the pathogenesis of smokers sperm alterations with a possible neuroendocrine mechanism [31]. Indeed, it has been demonstrated that nicotine and its metabolites are capable to cross the blood-testis barrier [32].

3.1. Effects on Testosterone Production

In vivo animal studies demonstrated that rat exposed to cigarette smoke show low testosterone elevation in response to human chorionic gonadotropin (hCG) stimulation compared to non-exposed rats [33]. The chronic administration of nicotine in male rats determined a reduction in testosterone and estradiol levels. This effect was counteracted by mecamylamine, an inhibitor of nicotine, proving that nicotine has a specific gonadotoxic effect [34]. The decreased testosterone levels seem to turn to normality after nicotine cessation, indicating a potential reversible effect of nicotine on Leydig cells function [35]. It has been demonstrated that nicotine and its metabolites inhibit multiple steps in testosterone biosynthesis. In rat Leydig cells, nicotine and cotinine produce a dose-dependent increase in progesterone levels and a dose-dependent decrease in testosterone concentration, by the inhibition of 17α-hydroxylase, 17,20-lyase, and 17-ketosteroid reductase [36]. Furthermore, nicotine exerts cytotoxic effects on mouse Leydig cells in a concentration- and time-dependent manner inducing apoptosis, as demonstrating by the increase in Bax (a pro-apoptotic protein) and caspase-3 expression and a decrease in Bcl-2 (an anti-apoptotic protein) expression [37].

Despite the evidence in animal studies of the cytotoxic effect of nicotine and cigarette smoke on Leydig cells, in male smokers a reduction of testosterone levels has not been clearly demonstrated. Conversely, most of the studies found higher testosterone levels in smokers than in non-smokers [38–42]. Higher testosterone and LH levels with higher LH/free testosterone ratio were found with increased smoking, hence authors hypothesized a compensated Leydig cell failure in smokers [40]. The concurrent increase in testosterone and LH levels was confirmed for current smokers of five or more cigarettes/day but not for smokers of less than five cigarettes/day [41]. Recently, a meta-analysis of 22 studies with a total of 13,317 men, confirmed that smokers show testosterone levels higher than non-smokers [43].

Since higher testosterone concentration should lower LH levels through the negative feedback exerted at central level, it has been postulated that tobacco alters hypothalamus-pituitary axis enhancing GnRH or LH release. Alternatively, it has been hypothesized that higher testosterone levels could be the basis of the smoking habit, favoring addiction to smoking, since men with higher testosterone levels tend to adopt more risky lifestyles [38,41]. Another mechanism that could contribute to testosterone rise in smokers is the inhibition of testosterone breakdown by nicotine's metabolites. Indeed, the uridine 5′-diphospho (UDP)-glucuronosyltransferase (UGT) enzyme superfamily catalyzes the glucuronidation of both testosterone and nicotine's metabolites; so, cotinine and trans-3′-hydroxycotinine can compete with testosterone for binding to the catalytic site and prevent androgen inactivation [43].

Nicotine at the mesolimbic level increases dopamine release, which in turn inhibits prolactin release from the hypophysis. Some studies showed lower prolactin levels in smokers than in non-smokers [38]; however, other studies reported higher prolactin levels in smokers [41]. This paradoxical effect could be explained by the action of endogenous opioids, released in response to nicotine, which could reduce dopamine release.

3.2. Effects on Spermatogenesis

The association between cigarette smoking and sperm concentration has been studied from the 80s. A first meta-analysis conducted in 1994 showed that smokers had a sperm density 13–17% lower than that of nonsmokers [44]. Subsequent studies confirmed this finding. Ten years later Künzle and colleagues found in smokers a decrease of about 15% in sperm density and of about 17% in total sperm count compared to nonsmokers [45]. Another study on over 2,500 men found an inverse dose–response relation between smoking and sperm count, with a 19% lower sperm concentration and a 29% lower total sperm count in heavy smokers compared to non-smokers [40]. Other studies failed to demonstrate a detrimental effect of cigarette smoking on sperm concentration [46,47] or found a trend for a reduction of sperm count with the increasing number of smoked cigarettes, without reaching statistical significance [48]. However, a more recent meta-analysis with a wider sample size confirmed that smoking is a risk factor for all sperm parameters, including sperm density and total count, in both infertile and healthy men [49]. Another meta-analysis was conducted in 2016, including only studies performed after the introduction of 2010 WHO manual for the laboratory evaluation of human semen. This meta-analysis involved a total of almost 6,000 participants, and found a reduced sperm count in smokers, with higher effect size in infertile men and in moderate/heavy smokers [50]. The latest meta-analysis, performed in 2019, evaluated sixteen studies including almost 11,000 infertile male participants subdivided in smokers and non-smokers and found that oligozoospermia is significantly more frequent in smokers with a relative risk of 1.29 [51].

It has been demonstrated in vitro that spermatozoa from healthy, non-smoker men incubated with cigarette smoke extract show an increase in phosphatidylserine externalization, an early apoptotic sign, and in DNA fragmentation, a late apoptotic sign, in a concentration- and time-dependent manner [52]. Similarly, the incubation of spermatozoa with increasing concentration of nicotine reduces the percentage of viable spermatozoa and increases the number of spermatozoa with altered chromatin compactness, or DNA fragmentation [53]. This finding indicates that nicotine itself is, at least in part, responsible for the detrimental effect of cigarette smoke on sperm. Indeed, nicotine and its major metabolites, cotinine and trans-3'-hydroxycotinine, are capable to cross the blood-testis barrier and their concentrations are similar or even higher in the seminal plasma than in the blood of smokers [32].

Nicotine binds to a class of ionotropic acetylcholine receptors, the nicotinic receptors (nAChR), made up of five subunits, whose expression has been demonstrated also on human spermatozoa. Since hexamethonium, the main antagonist for the neuronal nAChR, is able to reverse the detrimental effects of nicotine on non-conventional sperm parameters, including apoptotic signs, a possible neuroendocrine mechanism has been postulated for nicotine-related sperm damage [31]. In semen of non-smokers, only a homomeric nicotinic receptor consisting of five $\alpha 7$ subunits is present; however, it has been demonstrated that cigarette smoking may stimulate the expression of some other subunits, such as $\alpha 9$ subunit, that in pregnant smoker women is involved in the vasoconstriction, disepithelization, and apoptosis of the placenta. The aberrant expression of subunit different from $\alpha 7$ in semen could contribute to the functional alterations found in the spermatozoa of smokers and could represent a marker for smoking-related sperm damage [54].

In rats exposed to nicotine ultrastructural alterations of germ cells, peritubular structures, and Sertoli cells were found. These alterations include: thickening of the tunica propria; degeneration of junction between the Sertoli cells; irregular cristae and electron-dense matrix inside Sertoli cells' mitochondria; spermatids with altered cytoplasm-nucleus ratio, cytoplasmic electron-dense lipid droplets, and abnormal acrosome [55].

In addition to the gonadotoxic action of nicotine, reactive oxygen species (ROS) have been called into question as determinants of sperm damage in smokers. Indeed, smokers, have higher malondialdehyde, and protein carbonyls level (markers of oxidative stress), and lower glutathione, ascorbic acid, zinc, superoxide dismutase, catalase, and glutathione-S-Transferase than non-smokers [56]. Cadmium and lead levels in seminal plasma of smokers were correlated with the oxidative stress markers [57]. Erythroid 2-related factor 2 (NRF2), an antioxidative transcription activator that binds to antioxidant response elements in the promoter regions of target genes, could be implicated in the susceptibility of sperm damage induced by ROS in smokers. Indeed, the NRF2 rs6721961 TT genotype was found to be associated with lower sperm concentrations and sperm counts in heavy smokers [58].

4. Caffeine

Caffeine is a methylated xanthine, structurally similar to purine and uric acid, present in coffee, tea, soft drinks, and chocolate. One cup of coffee contains about 137 mg of caffeine, a cup of tea 47 mg, a bottle or can of caffeinated soft drinks (i.e., cola) about 46 mg, a serving of chocolate about 7 mg [59]. Caffeine stimulates heart contraction and rate, dilates blood vessels by relaxing smooth muscles, increases the secretion of catecholamine, increases diuresis, enhances alertness and decreases drowsiness and fatigue. It is able to cross the blood-testicular barrier and it is found in the same concentrations in blood and semen [60]. For these reasons, its effects on reproductive function have been investigated.

4.1. Effects on Testosterone Production

In a study of more than 2,500 men, no statistically significant association was found between caffeine intake and reproductive hormones [61]. However, in other studies caffeine consumption was positively associated with total [39,62] or bioavailable testosterone [63].

In animal models, caffeine induces a stress-like hormonal response. The acute treatment with high doses of caffeine caused in male rats a rise above control values in plasma concentrations of corticosterone, progesterone, testosterone, and noradrenaline [64]. Prolonged treatment for up to 30 days determined a significant increase in serum testosterone and a significant decrease in serum luteinizing hormone and follicle-stimulating hormone (FSH) levels [65].

4.2. Effects on Spermatogenesis

The evidence about a putative detrimental effect of caffeine on sperm production is controversial. Most of the studies showed no significant differences in sperm concentration in relation to caffeine intake [59,61,62,66–68]. Only cola soft drinks consumption has been associated with lower sperm count and concentration, but this effect is not directly related to caffeine because its content is much lower than in coffee [61]. However, an intake of more than 700 mg/d caffeine has been associated with a decreased fecundability rate both in men than in women [67], and a paternal intake of more than 272 mg/d has been associated with a decreased live birth rate in intracytoplasmic sperm injection (ICSI) cycles [59].

A recent systematic review of 28 studies and about 20,000 men confirmed that caffeine intake does not influence sperm count and concentration. However, data meta-analysis was not performed because of the extreme heterogeneity in exposure measurement (i.e., weekly intake of coffee alone or of different sources of caffeine), study design, and studied outcomes [25]. The single existing meta-analysis included only two studies and concluded for no statistically significant effects of coffee consumption on sperm density [49].

An animal study showed that Wistar rats orally treated with caffeine for 30 days have a decreased sperm count which does not ameliorate after caffeine withdrawal. Histological sections of the testis in treated rats showed subcapsular and interstitial congestion [65].

Caffeine acts as an antagonist of adenosine receptors. Adenosine receptors are also present in Sertoli cells where they seem to promotes the production of lactate, the preferred metabolic substrate of germ cells [69]. It has been demonstrated that the incubation of Sertoli cells with low-moderate doses of caffeine enhances lactate production and increases the expression of GLUT1 and GLUT3. However, at high concentration caffeine exerts on Sertoli cells a pro-oxidant effect [69].

5. Cannabis

Extract from Cannabis sativa, commonly referred to as marijuana, is the most widely used illegal drug in many countries. The major psychoactive substance contained in cannabis, Δ9-tetrahydrocannabinol (THC), is able to interact with cannabinoid receptors CB1 and CB2, belonging to the superfamily of G-protein coupled receptors. In humans, CB1 is localized in nervous system and other tissues, including reproductive system (ovary, uterine endometrium in women, testis and vas deferens in men), while CB2 is found predominantly in immune cells but also in Sertoli cells [70]. The endogenous ligands for cannabinoid receptors are the endocannabinoids produced and released on-demand by neurons and peripheral cells. The main endocannabinoids are anandamide and 2-arachidonoylglycerol [71]. The endocannabinoid system is involved in the regulation of reproductive function [72]. For these reasons, the effects of cannabis on male reproductive function have been investigated for almost 50 years, leading to contrasting results.

5.1. Effects on Testosterone Production

Since 1970s, a dose-related decrease in testosterone levels has been demonstrated in chronic marijuana smokers [73]. In acute administration, plasma LH was significantly depressed and cortisol was significantly elevated after smoking marijuana, indicating that cannabis decreases testosterone levels with a central mechanism [74]. Other studies failed to demonstrate statistically significant differences in plasma testosterone levels between occasional and chronic marijuana smokers [75], between occasional smokers and controls [76], or between daily cannabis users and controls [77]. A recent population study on over 1,500 U.S. men found no differences in serum testosterone levels among ever users of marijuana compared to never users. However, testosterone concentrations were higher in men with more recent marijuana use, especially in men aged 18–29 [78]. A study on over 1,200 young healthy men reported, similarly to tobacco smokers, an increase in testosterone levels in marijuana smokers [79]. A recent systematic review on 15 clinical studies and 21 animal/in vitro studies concluded for a not significant relationship between long-term cannabis consumption and alteration of the hypothalamic–pituitary–testicular axis hormones [80].

Despite these conflicting data, an inhibitory action of THC at central level is plausible since it has been demonstrated that CB1 receptors are present both at pituitary (expecially in lactotrophs and gonadotrophs) and hypothalamic (in GnRH neurons) level. Endocannabinoids depress the pituitary secretion of thyroid-stimulating hormone (TSH), LH, growth hormone (GH), and prolactin, and the hypothalamic GnRH release in rats [81]. Specifically, the CB1 receptor agonist anandamide suppresses LH and testosterone secretion [82]. In vitro, it has been demonstrated that endocannabinoids inhibit gamma-aminobutyric acid (GABA) A receptors drive in GnRH neurons, determining a decrease in GnRH neuron firing rate [83].

However, a direct effect of THC in testis has also been demonstrated in animal models. In rats, acute and chronic administration of THC significantly depressed testosterone formation in testis microsomes [84]. In in vitro studies, murine Leydig cells incubated with THC produced less testosterone in response to hCG and dibutyryl-cAMP [85]. Furthermore, a reduced expression of LH receptor on testis and a reduced activity of testicular 3β-hydroxysteroid dehydrogenase has been demonstrated in mice fed with a preparation containing cannabis [86].

5.2. Effects on Spermatogenesis

Parallel to the reduction of testosterone levels, a higher prevalence of oligozoospermia has been found in marijuana smokers since the 70s. Kolodny and colleagues found oligozoospermia in 35% of men who used marihuana without other drugs at least four days a week for a minimum of six months [73]. In a study on more than 1,200 healthy young men, the Authors found a lower sperm concentration and a lower total sperm count among men smoking marijuana more than once per week. The concomitant use of other recreational drugs was associated with a further worsening of sperm production [79]. Other studies failed to demonstrate a decrease in sperm count in marijuana smokers [87]. A recent systematic review of seven clinical studies and 23 animal/in vitro studies concluded that cannabis consumption exerts a negative impact on semen parameters, but it considered also the alteration of sperm motility and morphology that is not an argument of our review [80].

It has been demonstrated that endocannabinoids at male reproductive level inhibit acrosome reaction and sperm capacitation, and induce programmed cell death in Sertoli cells (effect counteracted by FSH) [71]. Since clinical studies on humans are not feasible for ethical reasons, most of the studies on spermatogenesis were carried on animals and demonstrated a detrimental effect of THC on germ cells. For example, daily administration of cannabis extract in dogs for one month produced a complete arrest of spermatogenesis, with extensive fibrosis and exfoliation of the seminiferous elements [88]. Regressive changes have also been demonstrated in the testes of mice fed with bhang, an Indian edible preparation of cannabis, for over 30 days [86]. The chronic administration of HU210, a synthetic analogue of THC and potent agonist of CB1 and CB2 receptors, determined in male rats a significant reduction in sperm count and daily sperm production, and a reduction in the number of Sertoli cells. No significant differences were observed after acute treatment [89]. Conversely, a recent study conducted on mice treated with a daily dose of 10 mg/kg THC for 30 days found no changes in testis weight nor alterations in spermatogenesis and sperm concentration. Moreover, the morphology of Sertoli and Leydig cells was normal, and apoptosis - evaluated with TUNEL test - was not different between the two groups [90].

6. Cocaine

Cocaine is an alkaloid obtained from the leaves of many species of the Erythroxylaceae family. It is a powerful local anesthetic, it alters thermoregulation and exerts stimulating effects on cardiovascular system, central and peripheral nervous system [91]. Cocaine abuse and dependence are very frequent, especially in Western countries. However, the relationship between cocaine intake and male reproductive function has not been extensively studied. In infertile male population, a low prevalence of cocaine use (<1%) has been reported, but men consuming cocaine are more likely to use other illicit drugs and substances (e.g., alcohol, tobacco) which may negatively impact their reproductive function [92].

6.1. Effects on Testosterone Production

Increase in LH, adrenocorticotropin hormone (ACTH), and cortisol, decrease in prolactin e unchanged testosterone levels have been found in men after intravenous low-dose cocaine injection (0.2–0.4 mg/kg) [93,94]. Conversely, in men who chronically use cocaine, lower free testosterone concentrations have been found, while gonadotropins did not differ compared to nonusers [95]. Furthermore, some cases of cocaine-induced panhypopituitarism have been described: intranasal cocaine abuse can cause pituitary infarction [96] or the production of human neutrophil elastase-anti-neutrophil cytoplasmic antibodies (HNE-ANCA), leading to a pituitary inflammatory process [97].

Regarding evidence on animals, a biphasic effect on the testosterone concentration has been found in rats following intraperitoneal injections of high doses of cocaine: testosterone initially raised and then dropped quickly [98]. In another study, male Wistar rats treated with intraperitoneal injections of low doses of cocaine showed an increase in testosterone concentration and unaltered LH levels. The same effect was not demonstrated with high doses of cocaine [91]. Similarly, the chronic administration of cocaine (15 mg/kg for 100 days) in rats did not induce changes in testosterone, FSH and LH levels [99]. In male Rhesus monkeys, a single injection of low dose cocaine caused a rapid increase in LH levels, while testosterone concentration did not change. The Authors hypothesized that LH release following cocaine injection was due to a burst of hypothalamic GnRH [100].

6.2. Effects on Spermatogenesis

Since the 1990s, the association between oligozoospermia and cocaine consumption has been investigated. Bracken and colleagues found an odds ratio of 2.1 of having sperm counts $<20 \times 10^6$ mL in men who referred cocaine use [101].

In male rats repeated intraperitoneal injections of low and high doses of cocaine produced a decline in the number of normal seminiferous tubules of respectively 50% and 40%, and an increase in regressive tubules of 50% and 60%. Testis weight was not significantly reduced after treatment; however, the testicular volume decreased after high doses of cocaine. The main cytological changes found in spermatogonia, spermatids, and Sertoli cells were lipid droplets, vacuoles and giant mitochondria [91]. Effects of long-term cocaine administration on spermatogenesis were similar: peripubertal rats treated for 100 days with cocaine showed a reduced mean diameter of seminiferous tubules and thickness of the germinal epithelium. The number of spermatids also decreased. These findings indicate a significant toxic action on spermatogenesis, that Authors attributed to the ischemic effect of cocaine. Indeed, cocaine, enhancing norepinephrine and epinephrine release, induces intense vasoconstriction [99]. It has been demonstrated that cocaine chronic administration increases germ cell apoptosis, evaluated by TUNEL assay, of about 25%. Since ROS activate apoptosis and are generated during the metabolization of cocaine and during reperfusion injury, they have been implicated in the cocaine-induced programmed cell death [102,103].

7. Amphetamine, Methamphetamine, and MDMA (Ecstasy)

Amphetamine is a drug derived from phenethylamine with the addition of an α-methyl group that protects it against metabolism by monoamine oxidase. It stimulates the release of monoamines (i.e., dopamine and noradrenaline) in central nervous system and it has been used since the 1930s in the treatment of psychiatric disorders [104]. It is still employed in the U.S. and in some European countries in the management of Attention Deficit/Hyperactivity Disorder (ADHD); however, for its euphoric and stimulant effects, it is also taken for recreational purposes. Methamphetamine is obtained from the methylation of amphetamine which confers it greater psychostimulant activity. It is also known with the street names Speed and Meth Crystal and it is often abused for recreational purpose. 3,4-Methylenedioxymethamphetamine (MDMA), commonly known as Ecstasy, is a synthetic amphetamine, with serotonin and dopamine-releasing properties. It has several stimulating and inhibiting effects on central and peripheral nervous system (i.e., euphoria, increased energy, insomnia, enhanced sensory perception; attention and memory deficit, reduction of psychomotor speed and executive cognitive function); furthermore, it alters circadian rhythms and thermoregulation, causing hyperthermia. It is the entactogen molecule par excellence since it is able to produce feelings of empathy [105]. Amphetamines have demonstrated, in experimental settings, several effects on testicular function, as summarized below. However, studies on humans are not available.

7.1. Effects on Testosterone Production

In vivo and in vitro studies demonstrated that amphetamine decreases testosterone production and increases the generation of testicular cyclic AMP in rats. Also hCG-stimulated testosterone release was reduced in rats following a single intravenous injection of amphetamine, while plasma LH levels did not change. Authors hypothesized that amphetamine could act directly and dose-dependently on Leydig cells, and that the activation of adenylate cyclase could be responsible for the inhibition of testosterone production after amphetamine administration [106]. The same Authors demonstrated subsequently that in Leydig cells amphetamine decreases the activity of the steroidogenic enzymes 3b-hydroxysteroid dehydrogenase, P450c17, and 17-ketosteroid reductase, and attenuates Ca^{2+} influx through L-type Ca^{2+} channel [107]. Another study evaluated the effects of amphetamine on steroidogenesis in MA-10 mouse Leydig tumor cells, which produce progesterone as the major steroid instead of testosterone in response to hCG. Contrary to previous studies, the Authors demonstrated a stimulatory action of amphetamine, which directly enhanced hCG-induced progesterone production in cells by increasing the activity of the P450scc enzyme. No effects on the activity enzymes 3b-hydroxysteroid dehydrogenase was found [108].

In an in vivo study, a single intraperitoneal administration of methamphetamine exerted a biphasic effect on testosterone production in mice: serum testosterone concentrations initially decreased and then increased, reaching a level higher than basal after 48 hours. The Author postulated that, similarly to amphetamine, methamphetamine could decrease testosterone production acting at testicular level [109]. In another study, rats chronically treated with high doses of methamphetamine exhibited lower testosterone levels compared to controls [110]. An increase in testicular GABA concentration has also been reported in methamphetamine treated rats [111]. Since GABA is involved in the proliferation of Leydig cells and testosterone production, Authors hypothesized that the increase in GABA concentration could represent a compensatory response to the detrimental effects of methamphetamine on Leydig cells [111].

It has been demonstrated that MDMA suppresses the hypothalamic-pituitary-gonadal axis in male rats. Following acute or chronic MDMA administration, adult male Sprague-Dawley rats showed lower expression of GnRH mRNA and decreased serum testosterone concentrations compared to controls. LH, progesterone, and estradiol concentrations were not affected, suggesting a diminished drive from hypothalamic GnRH neurons as the cause of the hypothalamic-pituitary-gonadal axis inhibition [112]. Since both dopamine and serotonin receptors are expressed in the preoptic area, where GnRH cell bodies allocate, these two neurotransmitters are probably implicated in the inhibition of GnRH mRNA expression [112]. Conversely, another study, in which MDMA was administered to male rats subcutaneously during 12 weeks one a day for three consecutive days a week, simulating human weekend associated consumption, failed to demonstrate any effects of MDMA on the hypothalamus-pituitary-gonadal axis hormones [113].

7.2. Effects on Spermatogenesis

In has been demonstrated that methamphetamine induces apoptosis in murine testicular germ cells: in mice treated with increasing intra-peritoneal doses of methamphetamine a dose-dependent percentage rise of the apoptotic tubules was detected by TUNEL. Histological changes found in the murine testis include vacuolization of spermatogonia and derangement of cell layers [114]. These findings were confirmed by another study demonstrating that methamphetamine administration decreases significantly cell proliferation and increases apoptosis in both rats spermatogonia and primary spermatocytes, altering proliferation/apoptosis ratio [115]. Another confirmation came from the study of Nudmamud-Thanoi and Thanoi, were rats treated acutely and sub-acutely with methamphetamine showed an increase in TUNEL-positive cells in seminiferous tubules and a parallel reduction in epididymal sperm count [116]. In a more recent study, rats receiving 5 ml/kg intraperitoneal methamphetamine for 7 and 14 days showed a significant decrease in the number of spermatogonia, primary and secondary spermatocytes, and in spermatogenesis indices (tubular differentiation index, spermiogenesis index, repopulation index, and mean seminiferous tubules diameter) compared with controls [117].

Apoptosis in germ cells could be induced by hydroxyl radical formation, overproduction of serotonin or methamphetamine-induced testicular thermic rise [115]. In rats chronically treated with high doses of methamphetamine a significant decrease in GSH/GSSG ratio was recorded, indicating oxidative stress. Antioxidant enzymes (superoxide dismutase, catalase, and glutathione peroxidase) initially declined and then returned to normal, suggesting an adaptive response to scavenge ROS produced during methamphetamine metabolism. In parallel, a decreased expression of Bcl2 and increased levels of cleaved caspase-3 were found, indicating the activation of apoptosis. The Authors also reported a reduced epididymal sperm count in treated rats [110]. Methamphetamine seems also to reduce in male rats the expression of progesterone and estrogen receptors [116]. These receptors are normally expressed both in germ cells and in Sertoli cells and seem to play a role in germ cells proliferation and differentiation during development, inhibition of apoptosis, spermiogenesis, and sperm capacitation [118]. Finally, increased GABA concentrations have been found in rat testicular tissue after methamphetamine administration. Since GABA activity can suppress the proliferation of spermatogonial stem cells, the increase in its concentration could lead to alteration of proliferation/apoptosis ratio [111].

Also MDMA is able to cause histological alterations in rat testis. After subcutaneously MDMA administrations one a day for three consecutive days a week over a 12 weeks period, mild tubular degeneration and interstitial edema were observed in rat testicular tissue. The Comet assay showed a significant dose-related increase in sperm DNA damage; however, surprisingly, there was a significant enhancement of sperm count and a decrease in spermatids count in treated rats [113]. In another study conducted on rats, MDMA significantly increased the number of apoptotic TUNEL-positive cells in both germinal epithelium and Leydig cells, while germinal epithelium thickness and diameter of the tubules decreased. In parallel, an increase in body temperature and in immunoreactivity of heat shock protein 70 (HSP70) was observed [119]. Since testes are sensitive to temperature and HSP are produced in response to thermic stress to stop caspase activation and inhibit the apoptotic process, the Authors hypothesized that MDMA-induced hyperthermia could activate apoptosis in rat testicular tissue [119].

8. Opioids

Opioids are derived from opium, extracted from the seed pod of the opium poppy (Papaver somniferum). They include opium alkaloids, such as morphine, and synthetic derivatives, such as codeine and heroin. They have the ability to bind with three main classes of receptors - mu (μ), delta (δ), and kappa (κ) - belonging to the superfamily of G-protein coupled receptors, which usually interact with three major classes of endogenous opioid peptides (endorphins, enkephalins, and dynorphins) [120]. The endogenous opioids are physiologically implicated in the regulation of several functions: motor, immune, gastrointestinal, cardiovascular, neuroendocrine, cognitive, and, more notoriously, nociceptive function. Opioid analgesics, such as oxycodone, hydrocodone, propoxyphen, fentanyl, and methadone are frequently prescribed in muscular-skeletal and rheumatological conditions because they are effective in reducing pain, inexpensive and long-lasting. However, their potential risk for addiction is well known [120]. Opioid receptor antagonists, such as naloxone and naltrexone, are clinically used to reverse the effects of opioid overdose. The inhibitory effects of opioids on testosterone production are widely known; while effects on spermatogenesis are still controversial.

8.1. Effects on Testosterone Production

Opioid-induced androgen deficiency (OPIAD) is nowadays a recognized syndrome characterized by decreased levels of testosterone, reduced libido and muscle mass, fatigue, and osteopenia [121]. A cross-sectional study examined the prevalence of opioid use in the last 30 days in almost 5000 men and women aged 17 years and older from the general population. Testosterone levels of opioid-exposed were compared with those of non-exposed subjects. The Author found an overall OR = 1.40 of having low testosterone levels in opioid-exposed subjects. The most commonly used opioids were hydrocodone, oxycodone, and tramadol [122].

The inhibitory effects of opioid drugs on hypothalamic–pituitary–testicular axis have been known for over 40 years [123]. Endogenous and exogenous opioids inhibit hypothalamic GnRH secretion, disrupting its normal pulsatility and leading to decreased LH levels. As a consequence of reduced GnRH secretion, LH and therefore testosterone levels decrease, determining hypogonadotropic hypogonadism. The FSH levels would seem to be less affected by opioids administration, in both animals and men [120]. Hyperprolactinemia may contribute to opioids central inhibitory activity. Indeed, acute administration of opioids increases prolactin levels in both human and animal models, while their chronic administration could have variable effects on prolactin secretion based on the type of opioid used [120].

Men treated with long-term intrathecal opioid administration exhibit lower LH, serum testosterone and free androgen index than controls [124]. Low levels of total and free testosterone and high levels of SHBG have been also reported in heroin-addicted men [125,126] and in men consuming sustained-action oral opioids for control of non-malignant pain [127]. In a study on opium-addicted Iranian men, mean serum levels for LH, total, and free testosterone were significantly lower than in controls [128].

It has been hypothesized that not all opioids exert the same effect on testosterone production. Indeed, buprenorphine, a partial µ-opioid receptor agonist and pure antagonist at the κ-opioid receptor, used to treat opioid dependence, affects fewer testosterone levels than methadone [129–131]. Contrary to this hypothesis, a meta-analysis including 12 studies on men found a difference in testosterone levels of 165 ng/dL in men using opioids compared to controls, with no significant differences between the different types of opioids. The Authors concluded that all opioids suppress testosterone; however, only one study on buprenorphine was included in the meta-analysis [132]. It has also been demonstrated that long-acting opioids induce more frequently hypogonadism than short-acting opioids, probably for their prolonged inhibitory action on GnRH release [133].

Several studies demonstrated the inhibitory effects of opioids on the hypothalamic-pituitary-gonadal axis also in animal models. Four days of treatment with morphine determined in rat hypothalamus a marked decrease in GnRH mRNA levels, indicating that opioids inhibit the biosynthesis of the neuropeptide [134]. In vivo and in vitro studies demonstrated that methadone inhibits the dopamine-stimulated release of GnRH in rats [135]. Following morphine injection, testosterone levels decreased in rats dose-dependently and this effect was counteracted by the opioid antagonists naltrexone and naloxone [136]. Rats intraperitoneally injected for 30 days with tramadol hydrochloride, a widely used analgesic drug which binds to µ-opioid receptors more weakly than morphine, exhibited lower LH, FSH and testosterone levels than controls after treatment [137]. Another study found reduced LH levels in rats chronically treated with morphine, but FSH and testosterone levels did not significantly differ compared to controls. However, in this study the morphine administered dose was relatively low [138].

8.2. Effects on Spermatogenesis

It has been demonstrated that human spermatozoa express µ-, δ-, and κ- opioid receptors, located in the head, in the middle region, and in the tail of the sperm [139]. In a study conducted in Iran, where opium consumption is relatively common in the male population, opium-addicted men showed more frequently oligozoospermia than controls. Furthermore, they exhibited lower antioxidant activity and higher sperm DNA fragmentation index compared to healthy age-matched male volunteers [128].

Rats chronically treated with tramadol exhibited histological degenerative changes in the seminiferous tubules, in Sertoli cells and in Leydig cells: tubules showed a decrease in mean diameter and epithelial height, shrinkage, separation of tubular basement membrane, and disorganization and vacuolization of spermatogenic layers; Sertoli cell presented vacuolation, huge lipid droplets and disrupted junctions; Leydig cells had euchromatic nuclei and dilated smooth endoplasmic reticulum [137]. The Authors suggested that regressive histological changes following tramadol administration were linked to opioid-induced testosterone deprivation [137].

Recently, increased caspase-3 and decreased anti-apoptotic protein Bcl-2 expression have been described in rats chronically treated with tramadol. Authors hypothesized that the apoptotic process was induced by oxidative stress since malonldialdehyde levels were increased, while the antioxidant enzymes activity was decreased in treated rats [140]. Interestingly, tramadol withdrawal improved but did not normalize apoptotic changes in testicular tissues, indicating permanent opioid-induced damage [140].

Another study failed to demonstrate a reduction of seminiferous tubules diameter in rats chronically treated with morphine, even if sperm count was three times lower in treated rats than controls. Also the distribution of Leydig and Sertoli cells did not differ from the two groups. However, the dose of morphine administered was on average lower than in the other studies [138]. These findings are partially in agreement with a study of Cicero and colleagues, where morphine treatment did not induce histological changes in the testis of rats treated with morphine. However, in this study – were morphine was administered at higher dosage but only for 14 days – also sperm count was normal [141]. These results could indicate that morphine exerts less gonadotoxic effects than other synthetic opioids, or that high dose and duration of treatment are both needed to reveal the detrimental effects of morphine on testis histology and function.

9. Anabolic-Androgenic Steroids

Anabolic-androgenic steroids (AAS) are the most used drugs by athletes, amateur sportsmen, and body-builders all over the world to improve sports performance and/or physical appearance. The global lifetime prevalence rate of their use is 6.4% for males [142]. At least 30 different AAS exist, including testosterone, its 17α-alkyl-derivates (e.g., oxandrolone, stanozolol), its 17β-ester-derivates (e.g., nandrolone, testosterone esters), and its precursors (androstenedione, dehydroepiandrosterone) [143]. The detrimental effect of AAS on endogenous androgens production and spermatogenesis are widely known and below summarized.

9.1. Effects on Testosterone Production

The AAS-induced hypogonadism is a widespread phenomenon. Indeed, in men younger than 50 years, the most common etiology of profound hypogonadism, defined as testosterone 50 ng/dl or less, is just the previous assumption of AAS [144]. Anabolic-androgenic steroids suppress gonadotropin release from the pituitary gland by a negative feedback mechanism, exerted on both pituitary gland and hypothalamic GnRH-releasing cells. This results in a down-regulation of gonadotropins and a decreased secretion of endogenous steroids [143]. Therefore, while during administration abusers may exhibit high androgen levels, they became hypogonadal following AAS discontinuation, especially after prolonged use.

A recent systematic review and meta-analysis revealed that long-term AAS use results in prolonged hypogonadotropic hypogonadism. In almost all studies included in the meta-analysis, LH and FSH serum levels decreased during AAS use and progressively increased, until returning to the basal levels, following AAS withdrawal. Conversely, testosterone blood concentration, which decreased during AAS abuse, remained lower compared to baseline following 16 weeks of AAS discontinuation [145].

The recovery of hypothalamus-pituitary-testicular axis can take from a few weeks to over a year after AAS withdrawal [146,147]. However, a recent cross-sectional case-control study, involving 37 current AAS abusers, 33 former AAS abusers who ceased steroids for at least 1.7 years, and 30 healthy controls, found that almost one-third of former AAS abusers had total testosterone levels below 12.1 nmol/L, indicating persistent hypogonadism [148]. Indeed, it has been demonstrated in animal studies that a permanent depletion of Leydig cells may occur following AAS administration. A reduction of interstitial cells' number has been reported in testicular tissue of pre-pubertal and adult male rats treated with high doses of AAS. Differently from pre-pubertal animals, which obtained a complete recovery of the Leydig cells number following AAS withdrawal, in adult rats Leydig cells did not return to the control level, suggesting a long-lasting alteration [149].

9.2. Effects on Spermatogenesis

The AAS abuse leads to severe oligozoospermia up to azoospermia because the elevated levels of exogenous androgens inhibit, via a hypothalamic and pituitary negative feedback, gonadotropin and testosterone production. The lack of LH and the consequent functional arrest of Leydig cells determines a marked reduction of intratesticular testosterone, of which adequate concentrations are required to maintain normal spermatogenesis [150]. Furthermore, FSH, in physiological condition, stimulates Sertoli cell to secrete androgen binding protein that conveys testosterone in the lumen of seminiferous tubules. The lack of FSH due to AAS-induced suppression thus aggravates the intratesticular hypotestosteronemia and its consequences on spermatogenesis [151].

Several studies demonstrated that bodybuilders using AAS have a reduced sperm concentration and a higher prevalence of azoospermia compared to controls [152,153]. Current AAS abusers have smaller testicular volume than former AAS abusers and controls, and exhibit markedly decreased plasma gonadotropins, SHBG, 17-hydroxyprogesterone, serum anti-müllerian hormone (AMH) and inhibin B levels. Serum AMH and inhibin B are Sertoli cells biomarkers and low levels are suggestive of impaired spermatogenesis [148].

As for AAS-induced hypogonadotropic hypogonadism, the alteration of spermatogenesis are usually transient. An integrated multivariate time-to-event analysis of data from 30 studies including about 1,500 subjects who assumed AAS for male contraception, revealed that the median time for sperm to recover to 20 million per mL was 3.4 months. The probability of recovery to 20 million per mL was 67% within 6 months, 90% within 12 months, and 100% within 24 months [154]. Since AAS doses used for male contraception are significantly lower than those used for doping purposes, in abusers even longer time could be required to recover spermatogenesis. In any case, the recovery time depends on the individual characteristics of the subject. It has been hypothesized that men who do not obtain normal sperm concentration following AAS withdrawal, could have unknown fertility alterations before starting AAS consumption [155].

An increase in apoptotic processes has also been implicated in the pathogenesis of oligozoospermia following AAS treatment. In rats treated with nandrolone, a statistically significant decrease in testicular weight and in total epididymal sperm count was observed. Contextually, an increase in TUNEL-positive cells and caspase-3 enzyme activity was recorded, indicating the activation of apoptosis [151].

10. Conclusions

Surely, substance abuse can contribute to the increased prevalence of hypogonadism observed in Western countries. However, not all abused drugs have a significant negative impact on testicular function.

A low-moderate alcohol intake would seem not to impair reproductive function [22]. Conversely, in heavy drinkers and alcoholic men, both testosterone production and spermatogenesis are altered with multiple mechanisms. Alcohol inhibits some stages of steroidogenesis, increases the conversion of testosterone in estradiol inducing the enzyme aromatase, suppresses β-LH gene expression and protein release from the pituitary gland, and inhibits hypothalamic GnRH secretion through the increase in β-endorphin-like peptides [9–11,14,15]. Furthermore, it has been demonstrated that alcohol induces testicular atrophy and histological regressive changes, enhances the production of ROS, and reduces the anti-oxidant testicular defenses [8,10,29].

Regarding tobacco, it has been demonstrated that both cigarette smoke extract and nicotine increase apoptotic markers in sperm [52,53]. Indeed, four meta-analyses have confirmed that smoking is a risk factor for oligozoospermia [44,49–51]. Testicular damage is probably due to smoke-induced oxidative stress, but also a neuroendocrine mechanism of nicotine has been hypothesized [31]. Conversely, tobacco does not decrease testosterone levels in men; rather, it would seem to increase androgen concentrations with mechanisms not entirely clear [43].

Caffeine would not seem to reduce testosterone production nor spermatogenesis in men, even if a pro-oxidant effect has been described for very elevated dosage [69].

Despite animal studies showed a decreased testosterone production after exposition to cannabis, a clear relationship between marijuana use and hypogonadism has not been found in men. However, marijuana users have worse sperm parameters, including sperm total count and concentration, compared to controls in most studies [80].

Data about cocaine are few and contrasting. Overall, cocaine abuse seems not to reduce testosterone levels. However, an odds ratio of 2.1 of having low sperm concentration has been found in cocaine abusers [101]. Some Authors found histological regressive changes and apoptotic markers in both germ and Sertoli cells in rats treated with cocaine [91].

Data about the effects of amphetamines on human testicular function are lacking and those on animals are contrasting. Amphetamine, methamphetamine, and MDMA caused variably positive, negative and no effects on testosterone concentrations in rats [109,110,113]. Regarding spermatogenesis, amphetamines induce apoptosis in murine testicular germ cells [114]. Oxidative stress, overproduction of serotonin and GABA, thermic rise, and decreased expression of progesterone and estradiol receptors in testis have been called into question in the pathogenesis of testicular damage [111,116,119].

Opioids intake is a known cause of hypogonadotropic hypogonadism. Indeed, opioids are able to suppress the hypothalamic-pituitary-gonadal axis, with variable grade and intensity depending on the type of compound [120]. The effects on spermatogenesis are less clear. Only one study showed a higher prevalence of oligozoospermia in opium-addicted males [128]. In rats, histological changes, increased apoptosis, and oxidative stress have been described [137].

The inhibitory effects of AAS on testosterone production and spermatogenesis are also widely known. Anabolic-androgenic steroids exert negative feedback on both pituitary gland and hypothalamus, suppressing the release of gonadotropins and testosterone [143]. Testicular volume decreases and sperm production, no longer supported by adequate intratubular testosterone concentration, drops. These effects are usually reversible, even if a complete recovery of the axis can take more than one year. However, incomplete normalization of testosterone levels and sperm production following AAS withdrawal have also been described [148].

The main mechanisms by which substance abuse interferes with testosterone production and spermatogenesis are summarized in Figure 1 and in Table 1.

The effect of the concomitant abuse of more than one of the substances is unpredictable but often additive. The substance withdrawal in most cases leads to the resolution of the hypogonadism. Indeed, during the evaluation of the patient referring for hypogonadism, to investigate the use of illicit drugs and legal substances such as tobacco and alcohol is mandatory. Especially in younger men, when no organic causes of hypogonadism are detectable, substance abuse must be suspected and, eventually, the withdrawal must be recommended.

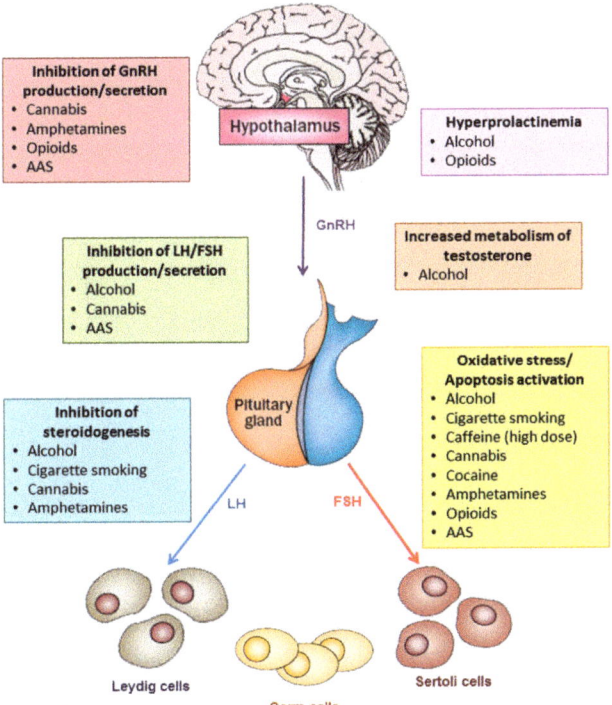

Figure 1. The main mechanisms by which substance/drug abuse may decrease testosterone levels and sperm production are: inhibition oh GnRH production/secretion, increase in prolactin levels, inhibition of gonadotropin production/secretion, inhibition of steroidogenesis, increase in testosterone metabolism, oxidative stress, induction of apoptosis. Abbreviations: AAS = anabolic-androgenic steroids, FSH = follicle-stimulating hormone; GnRH = gonadotropin-releasing hormone; LH = luteinizing hormone.

Table 1. Effects of each substance/drug on testosterone levels and sperm production, and main evidences of the pathophysiological mechanisms. ↑: increase in testosterone/sperm concentration; ↓: decrease in testosterone/sperm concentration; ↔: no effects on testosterone/sperm concentration; FSH: follicle-stimulating hormone; GABA: gamma-aminobutyric acid; GnRH: gonadotropin-releasing hormone; LH: luteinizing hormone; ROS: reactive oxygen species; StAR: steroidogenic acute regulatory protein

Substance	Effect on Testosterone	Hypothesized Mechanisms	Effect on Sperm Concentration	Hypothesized Mechanisms
Alcohol	↓	Suppression of β-LH gene expression [14] Prolactin increase after acute ingestion [9] Inhibition of 3β-hydroxysteroid dehydrogenase and 17-ketosteroid reductase [9] Suppressed expression of StAR via ROS [10] Induction of the enzyme aromatase [11] Enhanced GnRH or LH release [38,41]	↓	Induction of apoptosis [10] Pro-oxidant effect [29]
Cigarette smoking	↑	Inhibition of prolactin release [38] Competitive inhibition of testosterone glucuronidation [43]	↓	Induction of apoptosis [52,53] Pro-oxidant effect [56–58]
Caffeine	↑	Induction of a stress-like hormonal pattern [64] Inhibition of GnRH and LH in animal models [81,83] Reduced expression of LH receptor on testis in animal models [86]	↔	Pro-oxidant effect at very high doses [69]
Cannabis	↔	Reduced activity of testicular 3β-hydroxysteroid dehydrogenase in animal models [86]	↓	Induction of apoptosis [71]
Cocaine	↔	Panhypopituitarism for pituitary infarction or inflammation (case reports) [96,97]	↓	Testicular vasoconstriction and ischemia [99] Induction of apoptosis [102] Pro-oxidant effect (reperfusion injury) [103]
Amphetamines	↓	Decreased expression of GnRH mRNA [112] Activation of adenylate cyclase [106] Inhibition of 3b-hydroxysteroid dehydrogenase, P450c17, and 17-ketosteroid reductase [107] Reduced Ca²⁺ influx [107] Increased testicular GABA concentration [111]	↓	Induction of apoptosis [114–116] Pro-oxidant effect [110] Testicular thermic damage [119] Increased testicular serotonin concentration [115] Increased testicular GABA concentration [111] Reduced testicular expression of progesterone and estrogen receptors [116]
Opioids	↓	Inhibition of GnRH secretion [120,134] Hyperprolactinemia [120]	↓	Induction of apoptosis [128,140] Pro-oxidant effect [128–140]
Anabolic-androgenic steroids (AAS)	↓	Inhibition of GnRH secretion [143] Inhibition of LH and FSH secretion [145] Depletion of Leydig cells [149]	↓	Reduction of intra-testicular testosterone levels [150,151] Induction of apoptosis [151]

Author Contributions: S.L. conceived the idea and revised the manuscript. Y.D. wrote the manuscript. A.A., A.E.C., and R.A.C. performed the literature search and corrected syntax and typos.

Funding: This research received no external funding.

Conflicts of Interest: The authors declare no conflict of interest.

References

1. Bhasin, S.; Brito, J.P.; Cunningham, G.R.; Hayes, F.J.; Hodis, H.N.; Matsumoto, A.M.; Snyder, P.J.; Swerdloff, R.S.; Wu, F.C.; Yialamas, M.A. Testosterone Therapy in Men with Hypogonadism: An Endocrine Society Clinical Practice Guideline. *J. Clin. Endocrinol. Metab.* **2018**, *103*, 1715–1744. [CrossRef]
2. Travison, T.G.; Araujo, A.B.; O'Donnell, A.B.; Kupelian, V.; McKinlay, J.B. A population-level decline in serum testosterone levels in American men. *J. Clin. Endocrinol. Metab.* **2007**, *92*, 196–202. [CrossRef]
3. Andersson, A.M.; Jensen, T.K.; Juul, A.; Petersen, J.H.; Jørgensen, T.; Skakkebaek, N.E. Secular decline in male testosterone and sex hormone binding globulin serum levels in Danish population surveys. *J. Clin. Endocrinol. Metab.* **2007**, *92*, 4696–4705. [CrossRef]
4. Levine, H.; Jørgensen, N.; Martino-Andrade, A.; Mendiola, J.; Weksler-Derri, D.; Mindlis, I.; Pinotti, R.; Swan, S.H. Temporal trends in sperm count: A systematic review and meta-regression analysis. *Hum. Reprod. Update* **2017**, *23*, 646–659. [CrossRef] [PubMed]
5. Travison, T.G.; Araujo, A.B.; Hall, S.A.; McKinlay, J.B. Temporal trends in testosterone levels and treatment in older men. *Curr. Opin. Endocrinol. Diabetes Obes.* **2009**, *16*, 211–217. [CrossRef] [PubMed]
6. Durairajanayagam, D. Lifestyle causes of male infertility. *Arab J. Urol.* **2018**, *16*, 10–20. [CrossRef]
7. La Vignera, S.; Condorelli, R.A.; Balercia, G.; Vicari, E.; Calogero, A.E. Does alcohol have any effect on male reproductive function? A review of literature. *Asian J. Androl.* **2013**, *15*, 221–225. [CrossRef]
8. Van Thiel, D.H.; Gavaler, J.S.; Cobb, C.F.; Santucci, L.; Graham, T.O. Ethanol, a Leydig cell toxin: Evidence obtained in vivo and in vitro. *Pharmacol. Biochem. Behav.* **1983**, *18* (Suppl. 1), 317–323. [CrossRef]
9. Muthusami, K.R.; Chinnaswamy, P. Effect of chronic alcoholism on male fertility hormones and semen quality. *Fertil. Steril.* **2005**, *84*, 919–924. [CrossRef]
10. Jana, K.; Jana, N.; De, D.K.; Guha, S.K. Ethanol induces mouse spermatogenic cell apoptosis in vivo through over-expression of Fas/Fas-L, p53, and caspase-3 along with cytochrome c translocation and glutathione depletion. *Mol. Reprod. Dev.* **2010**, *77*, 820–833. [CrossRef]
11. Gordon, G.G.; Southren, A.L.; Vittek, J.; Lieber, C.S. The effect of alcohol ingestion on hepatic aromatase activity and plasma steroid hormones in the rat. *Metabolism* **1979**, *28*, 20–24. [CrossRef]
12. Burra, P.; Franklyn, J.A.; Ramsden, D.B.; Elias, E.; Sheppard, M.C. Severity of alcoholic liver disease and markers of thyroid and steroid status. *Postgrad. Med. J.* **1992**, *68*, 804–810. [CrossRef]
13. Ida, Y.; Tsujimaru, S.; Nakamaura, K.; Shirao, I.; Mukasa, H.; Egami, H.; Nakazawa, Y. Effects of acute and repeated alcohol ingestion on hypothalamic-pituitary-gonadal and hypothalamic-pituitary-adrenal functioning in normal males. *Drug Alcohol Depend.* **1992**, *31*, 57–64. [CrossRef]
14. Emanuele, M.A.; Emanuele, N.V. Alcohol's effects on male reproduction. *Alcohol Health Res. World* **1998**, *22*, 195–201. [PubMed]
15. Gianoulakis, C. Characterization of the effects of acute ethanol administration on the release of beta-endorphin peptides by the rat hypothalamus. *Eur. J. Pharmacol.* **1990**, *180*, 21–29. [CrossRef]
16. Pajarinen, J.T.; Karhunen, P.J. Spermatogenic arrest and 'Sertoli cell-only' syndrome–common alcohol-induced disorders of the human testis. *Int. J. Androl.* **1994**, *17*, 292–299. [CrossRef]
17. Pajarinen, J.; Karhunen, P.J.; Savolainen, V.; Lalu, K.; Penttilä, A.; Laippala, P. Moderate alcohol consumption and disorders of human spermatogenesis. *Alcohol. Clin. Exp. Res.* **1996**, *20*, 332–337. [CrossRef]
18. Anderson, R.A., Jr.; Willis, B.R.; Oswald, C. Spontaneous recovery from ethanol-induced male infertility. *Alcohol* **1985**, *2*, 479–484. [CrossRef]
19. Vicari, E.; Arancio, A.; Giuffrida, V.; D'Agata, R.; Calogero, A.E. A case of reversible azoospermia following withdrawal from alcohol consumption. *J. Endocrinol. Investig.* **2002**, *25*, 473–476. [CrossRef]
20. Sermondade, N.; Elloumi, H.; Berthaut, I.; Mathieu, E.; Delarouzière, V.; Ravel, C.; Mandelbaum, J. Progressive alcohol-induced sperm alterations leading to spermatogenic arrest, which was reversed after alcohol withdrawal. *Reprod. Biomed. Online* **2010**, *20*, 324–327. [CrossRef]

21. Guthauser, B.; Boitrelle, F.; Plat, A.; Thiercelin, N.; Vialard, F. Chronic excessive alcohol consumption and male fertility: A case report on reversible azoospermia and a literature review. *Alcohol Alcohol.* **2014**, *49*, 42–44. [CrossRef]
22. Jensen, T.K.; Swan, S.; Jørgensen, N.; Toppari, J.; Redmon, B.; Punab, M.; Drobnis, E.Z.; Haugen, T.B.; Zilaitiene, B.; Sparks, A.E.; et al. Alcohol and male reproductive health: A cross-sectional study of 8344 healthy men from Europe and the USA. *Hum. Reprod.* **2014**, *29*, 1801–1809. [CrossRef]
23. Jensen, T.K.; Gottschau, M.; Madsen, J.O.; Andersson, A.M.; Lassen, T.H.; Skakkebæk, N.E.; Swan, S.H.; Priskorn, L.; Juul, A.; Jørgensen, N. Habitual alcohol consumption associated with reduced semen quality and changes in reproductive hormones; a cross-sectional study among 1221 young Danish men. *BMJ Open* **2014**, *4*, e005462. [CrossRef]
24. Boeri, L.; Capogrosso, P.; Ventimiglia, E.; Pederzoli, F.; Cazzaniga, W.; Chierigo, F.; Dehò, F.; Montanari, E.; Montorsi, F.; Salonia, A. Heavy cigarette smoking and alcohol consumption are associated with impaired sperm parameters in primary infertile men. *Asian J. Androl.* **2019**. [CrossRef]
25. Ricci, E.; Al Beitawi, S.; Cipriani, S.; Candiani, M.; Chiaffarino, F.; Viganò, P.; Noli, S.; Parazzini, F. Semen quality and alcohol intake: A systematic review and meta-analysis. *Reprod. Biomed. Online* **2017**, *34*, 38–47. [CrossRef]
26. Ricci, E.; Noli, S.; Ferrari, S.; La Vecchia, I.; Cipriani, S.; De Cosmi, V.; Somigliana, E.; Parazzini, F. Alcohol intake and semen variables: Cross-sectional analysis of a prospective cohort study of men referring to an Italian Fertility Clinic. *Andrology* **2018**, *6*, 690–696. [CrossRef]
27. Savolainen, V.T.; Pjarinen, J.; Perola, M.; Penttilä, A.; Karhunen, P.J. Glutathione-S-transferase GST M1 "null" genotype and the risk of alcoholic liver disease. *Alcohol. Clin. Exp. Res.* **1996**, *20*, 1340–1345. [CrossRef]
28. Pajarinen, J.; Savolainen, V.; Perola, M.; Penttilä, A.; Karhunen, P.J. Glutathione S-transferase-M1 'null' genotype and alcohol-induced disorders of human spermatogenesis. *Int. J. Androl.* **1996**, *19*, 155–163. [CrossRef]
29. Condorelli, R.A.; Calogero, A.E.; Vicari, E.; La Vignera, S. Chronic consumption of alcohol and sperm parameters: Our experience and the main evidences. *Andrologia* **2015**, *47*, 368–379. [CrossRef]
30. Stabbert, R.; Dempsey, R.; Diekmann, J.; Euchenhofer, C.; Hagemeister, T.; Haussmann, H.J.; Knorr, A.; Mueller, B.P.; Pospisil, P.; Reininghaus, W.; et al. Studies on the contributions of smoke constituents, individually and in mixtures, in a range of in vitro bioactivity assays. *Toxicol. In Vitro* **2017**, *42*, 222–246. [CrossRef]
31. Condorelli, R.A.; La Vignera, S.; Giacone, F.; Iacoviello, L.; Mongioì, L.M.; Li Volti, G.; Barbagallo, I.; Avola, R.; Calogero, A.E. Nicotine Effects and Receptor Expression on Human Spermatozoa: Possible Neuroendocrine Mechanism. *Front. Physiol.* **2017**, *8*, 177. [CrossRef]
32. Pacifici, R.; Altieri, I.; Gandini, L.; Lenzi, A.; Pichini, S.; Rosa, M.; Zuccaro, P.; Dondero, F. Nicotine, cotinine, and trans-3-hydroxycotinine levels in seminal plasma of smokers: Effects on sperm parameters. *Ther. Drug Monit.* **1993**, *15*, 358–363. [CrossRef]
33. Yamamoto, Y.; Isoyama, E.; Sofikitis, N.; Miyagawa, I. Effects of smoking on testicular function and fertilizing potential in rats. *Urol. Res.* **1998**, *26*, 45–48. [CrossRef]
34. Kavitharaj, N.K.; Vijayammal, P.L. Nicotine administration induced changes in the gonadal functions in male rats. *Pharmacology* **1999**, *58*, 2–7. [CrossRef]
35. Oyeyipo, I.P.; Raji, Y.; Bolarinwa, A.F. Nicotine alters male reproductive hormones in male albino rats: The role of cessation. *J. Hum. Reprod. Sci.* **2013**, *6*, 40–44. [CrossRef]
36. Yeh, J.; Barbieri, R.L.; Friedman, A.J. Nicotine and cotinine inhibit rat testis androgen biosynthesis in vitro. *J. Steroid Biochem.* **1989**, *33*, 627–630. [CrossRef]
37. Kim, K.H.; Joo, K.J.; Park, H.J.; Kwon, C.H.; Jang, M.H.; Kim, C.J. Nicotine induces apoptosis in TM3 mouse Leydig cells. *Fertil. Steril.* **2005**, *83* (Suppl. 1), 1093–1099. [CrossRef]
38. Trummer, H.; Habermann, H.; Haas, J.; Pummer, K. The impact of cigarette smoking on human semen parameters and hormones. *Hum. Reprod.* **2002**, *17*, 1554–1559. [CrossRef]
39. Svartberg, J.; Midtby, M.; Bønaa, K.H.; Sundsfjord, J.; Joakimsen, R.M.; Jorde, R. The associations of age, lifestyle factors and chronic disease with testosterone in men: The Tromsø Study. *Eur. J. Endocrinol.* **2003**, *149*, 145–152. [CrossRef]
40. Ramlau-Hansen, C.H.; Thulstrup, A.M.; Aggerholm, A.S.; Jensen, M.S.; Toft, G.; Bonde, J.P. Is smoking a risk factor for decreased semen quality? A cross-sectional analysis. *Hum. Reprod.* **2007**, *22*, 188–196. [CrossRef]

41. Blanco-Muñoz, J.; Lacasaña, M.; Aguilar-Garduño, C. Effect of current tobacco consumption on the male reproductive hormone profile. *Sci. Total Environ.* **2012**, *426*, 100–105. [CrossRef]
42. Lotti, F.; Corona, G.; Vitale, P.; Maseroli, E.; Rossi, M.; Fino, M.G.; Maggi, M. Current smoking is associated with lower seminal vesicles and ejaculate volume, despite higher testosterone levels, in male subjects of infertile couples. *Hum. Reprod.* **2015**, *30*, 590–602. [CrossRef] [PubMed]
43. Zhao, J.; Leung, J.Y.; Lin, S.L.; Schooling, C.M. Cigarette smoking and testosterone in men and women: A systematic review and meta-analysis of observational studies. *Prev. Med.* **2016**, *85*, 1–10. [CrossRef] [PubMed]
44. Vine, M.F.; Margolin, B.H.; Morrison, H.I.; Hulka, B.S. Cigarette smoking and sperm density: A meta-analysis. *Fertil. Steril.* **1994**, *61*, 35–43.
45. Künzle, R.; Mueller, M.D.; Hänggi, W.; Birkhäuser, M.H.; Drescher, H.; Bersinger, N.A. Semen quality of male smokers and nonsmokers in infertile couples. *Fertil. Steril.* **2003**, *79*, 287–291. [CrossRef]
46. Pasqualotto, F.F.; Sobreiro, B.P.; Hallak, J.; Pasqualotto, E.B.; Lucon, A.M. Cigarette smoking is related to a decrease in semen volume in a population of fertile men. *BJU Int.* **2006**, *97*, 324–326. [CrossRef]
47. De Jong, A.M.; Menkveld, R.; Lens, J.W.; Nienhuis, S.E.; Rhemrev, J.P. Effect of alcohol intake and cigarette smoking on sperm parameters and pregnancy. *Andrologia* **2014**, *46*, 112–117. [CrossRef]
48. Gaur, D.S.; Talekar, M.S.; Pathak, V.P. Alcohol intake and cigarette smoking: Impact of two major lifestyle factors on male fertility. *Indian J. Pathol. Microbiol.* **2010**, *53*, 35–40. [CrossRef] [PubMed]
49. Li, Y.; Lin, H.; Li, Y.; Cao, J. Association between socio-psycho-behavioral factors and male semen quality: Systematic review and meta-analyses. *Fertil. Steril.* **2011**, *95*, 116–123. [CrossRef]
50. Sharma, R.; Harlev, A.; Agarwal, A.; Esteves, S.C. Cigarette Smoking and Semen Quality: A New Meta-analysis Examining the Effect of the 2010 World Health Organization Laboratory Methods for the Examination of Human Semen. *Eur. Urol.* **2016**, *70*, 635–645. [CrossRef]
51. Bundhun, P.K.; Janoo, G.; Bhurtu, A.; Teeluck, A.R.; Soogund, M.Z.S.; Pursun, M.; Huang, F. Tobacco smoking and semen quality in infertile males: A systematic review and meta-analysis. *BMC Public Health* **2019**, *19*, 36. [CrossRef]
52. Calogero, A.; Polosa, R.; Perdichizzi, A.; Guarino, F.; La Vignera, S.; Scarfia, A.; Fratantonio, E.; Condorelli, R.; Bonanno, O.; Barone, N.; et al. Cigarette smoke extract immobilizes human spermatozoa and induces sperm apoptosis. *Reprod. Biomed. Online* **2009**, *19*, 564–571. [CrossRef]
53. Condorelli, R.A.; La Vignera, S.; Giacone, F.; Iacoviello, L.; Vicari, E.; Mongioì, L.; Calogero, A.E. In vitro effects of nicotine on sperm motility and bio-functional flow cytometry sperm parameters. *Int. J. Immunopathol. Pharmacol.* **2013**, *26*, 739–746. [CrossRef]
54. Condorelli, R.A.; La Vignera, S.; Duca, Y.; Zanghi, G.N.; Calogero, A.E. Nicotine Receptors as a Possible Marker for Smoking-related Sperm Damage. *Protein Pept. Lett.* **2018**, *25*, 451–454. [CrossRef]
55. Aydos, K.; Güven, M.C.; Can, B.; Ergün, A. Nicotine toxicity to the ultrastructure of the testis in rats. *BJU Int.* **2001**, *88*, 622–626. [CrossRef]
56. Dai, J.B.; Wang, Z.X.; Qiao, Z.D. The hazardous effects of tobacco smoking on male fertility. *Asian J. Androl.* **2015**, *17*, 954–960. [CrossRef]
57. Kiziler, A.R.; Aydemir, B.; Onaran, I.; Alici, B.; Ozkara, H.; Gulyasar, T.; Akyolcu, M.C. High levels of cadmium and lead in seminal fluid and blood of smoking men are associated with high oxidative stress and damage in infertile subjects. *Biol. Trace Elem. Res.* **2007**, *120*, 82–91. [CrossRef]
58. Yu, B.; Chen, J.; Liu, D.; Zhou, H.; Xiao, W.; Xia, X.; Huang, Z. Cigarette smoking is associated with human semen quality in synergy with functional NRF2 polymorphisms. *Biol. Reprod.* **2013**, *89*, 5. [CrossRef]
59. Karmon, A.E.; Toth, T.L.; Chiu, Y.H.; Gaskins, A.J.; Tanrikut, C.; Wright, D.L.; Hauser, R.; Chavarro, J.E.; Earth Study Team. Male caffeine and alcohol intake in relation to semen parameters and in vitro fertilization outcomes among fertility patients. *Andrology* **2017**, *5*, 354–361. [CrossRef]
60. Beach, C.A.; Bianchine, J.R.; Gerber, N. The excretion of caffeine in the semen of men: Pharmacokinetics and comparison of the concentrations in blood and semen. *J. Clin. Pharmacol.* **1984**, *24*, 120–126. [CrossRef]
61. Jensen, T.K.; Swan, S.H.; Skakkebaek, N.E.; Rasmussen, S.; Jørgensen, N. Caffeine intake and semen quality in a population of 2554 young Danish men. *Am. J. Epidemiol.* **2010**, *171*, 883–891. [CrossRef]
62. Ramlau-Hansen, C.H.; Thulstrup, A.M.; Bonde, J.P.; Olsen, J.; Bech, B.H. Semen quality according to prenatal coffee and present caffeine exposure: Two decades of follow-up of a pregnancy cohort. *Hum. Reprod.* **2008**, *23*, 2799–2805. [CrossRef] [PubMed]

63. Ferrini, R.L.; Barrett-Connor, E. Sex hormones and age: A cross-sectional study of testosterone and estradiol and their bioavailable fractions in community-dwelling men. *Am. J. Epidemiol.* **1998**, *147*, 750–754. [CrossRef] [PubMed]
64. Pollard, I. Increases in plasma concentrations of steroids in the rat after the administration of caffeine: Comparison with plasma disposition of caffeine. *J. Endocrinol.* **1988**, *119*, 275–280. [CrossRef]
65. Oluwole, O.F.; Salami, S.A.; Ogunwole, E.; Raji, Y. Implication of caffeine consumption and recovery on the reproductive functions of adult male Wistar rats. *J. Basic Clin. Physiol. Pharmacol.* **2016**, *27*, 483–491. [CrossRef]
66. Oldereid, N.B.; Rui, H.; Purvis, K. Life styles of men in barren couples and their relationship to sperm quality. *Int. J. Fertil.* **1992**, *37*, 343–349. [PubMed]
67. Jensen, T.K.; Henriksen, T.B.; Hjollund, N.H.; Scheike, T.; Kolstad, H.; Giwercman, A.; Ernst, E.; Bonde, J.P.; Skakkebaek, N.E.; Olsen, J. Caffeine intake and fecundability: A follow-up study among 430 Danish couples planning their first pregnancy. *Reprod. Toxicol.* **1998**, *12*, 289–295. [CrossRef]
68. Sobreiro, B.P.; Lucon, A.M.; Pasqualotto, F.F.; Hallak, J.; Athayde, K.S.; Arap, S. Semen analysis in fertile patients undergoing vasectomy: Reference values and variations according to age, length of sexual abstinence, seasonality, smoking habits and caffeine intake. *Sao Paulo Med. J.* **2005**, *123*, 161–166. [CrossRef]
69. Dias, T.R.; Alves, M.G.; Bernardino, R.L.; Martins, A.D.; Moreira, A.C.; Silva, J.; Barros, A.; Sousa, M.; Silva, B.M.; Oliveira, P.F. Dose-dependent effects of caffeine in human Sertoli cells metabolism and oxidative profile: Relevance for male fertility. *Toxicology* **2015**, *328*, 12–20. [CrossRef]
70. Park, B.; McPartland, J.M.; Glass, M. Cannabis, cannabinoids and reproduction. *Prostaglandins Leukot. Essent. Fat. Acids* **2004**, *70*, 189–197. [CrossRef]
71. Battista, N.; Pasquariello, N.; Di Tommaso, M.; Maccarrone, M. Interplay between endocannabinoids, steroids and cytokines in the control of human reproduction. *J. Neuroendocrinol.* **2008**, *20* (Suppl. 1), 82–89. [CrossRef]
72. Du Plessis, S.S.; Agarwal, A.; Syriac, A. Marijuana, phytocannabinoids, the endocannabinoid system, and male fertility. *J. Assist. Reprod. Genet.* **2015**, *32*, 1575–1588. [CrossRef] [PubMed]
73. Kolodny, R.C.; Masters, W.H.; Kolodner, R.M.; Toro, G. Depression of plasma testosterone levels after chronic intensive marihuana use. *N. Engl. J. Med.* **1974**, *290*, 872–874. [CrossRef]
74. Cone, E.J.; Johnson, R.E.; Moore, J.D.; Roache, J.D. Acute effects of smoking marijuana on hormones, subjective effects and performance in male human subjects. *Pharmacol. Biochem. Behav.* **1986**, *24*, 1749–1754. [CrossRef]
75. Mendelson, J.H.; Kuehnle, J.; Ellingboe, J.; Babor, T.F. Plasma testosterone levels before, during and after chronic marihuana smoking. *N. Engl. J. Med.* **1974**, *291*, 1051–1055. [CrossRef]
76. Cushman, P., Jr. Plasma testosterone levels in healthy male marijuana smokers. *Am. J. Drug Alcohol Abus.* **1975**, *2*, 269–275. [CrossRef]
77. Friedrich, G.; Nepita, W.; André, T. Serum testosterone concentrations in cannabis and opiate users. *Beitr. Gerichtl. Med.* **1990**, *48*, 57–66. [PubMed]
78. Thistle, J.E.; Graubard, B.I.; Braunlin, M.; Vesper, H.; Trabert, B.; Cook, M.B.; McGlynn, K.A. Marijuana use and serum testosterone concentrations among U.S. males. *Andrology* **2017**, *5*, 732–738. [CrossRef] [PubMed]
79. Gundersen, T.D.; Jørgensen, N.; Andersson, A.M.; Bang, A.K.; Nordkap, L.; Skakkebæk, N.E.; Priskorn, L.; Juul, A.; Jensen, T.K. Association Between Use of Marijuana and Male Reproductive Hormones and Semen Quality: A Study Among 1215 Healthy Young Men. *Am. J. Epidemiol.* **2015**, *182*, 473–481. [CrossRef]
80. Rajanahally, S.; Raheem, O.; Rogers, M.; Brisbane, W.; Ostrowski, K.; Lendvay, T.; Walsh, T. The relationship between cannabis and male infertility, sexual health, and neoplasm: A systematic review. *Andrology* **2019**, *7*, 139–147. [CrossRef] [PubMed]
81. Fasano, S.; Meccariello, R.; Cobellis, G.; Chianese, R.; Cacciola, G.; Chioccarelli, T.; Pierantoni, R. The endocannabinoid system: An ancient signaling involved in the control of male fertility. *Ann. N. Y. Acad. Sci.* **2009**, *1163*, 112–124. [CrossRef]
82. Wenger, T.; Ledent, C.; Csernus, V.; Gerendai, I. The central cannabinoid receptor inactivation suppresses endocrine reproductive functions. *Biochem. Biophys. Res. Commun.* **2001**, *284*, 363–368. [CrossRef]
83. Farkas, I.; Kalló, I.; Deli, L.; Vida, B.; Hrabovszky, E.; Fekete, C.; Moenter, S.M.; Watanabe, M.; Liposits, Z. Retrograde endocannabinoid signaling reduces GABAergic synaptic transmission to gonadotropin-releasing hormone neurons. *Endocrinology* **2010**, *151*, 5818–5829. [CrossRef] [PubMed]
84. List, A.; Nazar, B.; Nyquist, S.; Harclerode, J. The effects of delta9-tetrahydrocannabinol and cannabidiol on the metabolism of gonadal steroids in the rat. *Drug Metab. Dispos.* **1977**, *5*, 268–272.

85. Jakubovic, A.; McGeer, E.G.; McGeer, P.L. Effects of cannabinoids on testosterone and protein synthesis in rat testis Leydig cells in vitro. *Mol. Cell. Endocrinol.* **1979**, *15*, 41–50. [CrossRef]
86. Banerjee, A.; Singh, A.; Srivastava, P.; Turner, H.; Krishna, A. Effects of chronic bhang (cannabis) administration on the reproductive system of male mice. *Birth Defects Res. B Dev. Reprod. Toxicol.* **2011**, *92*, 195–205. [CrossRef]
87. Close, C.E.; Roberts, P.L.; Berger, R.E. Cigarettes, alcohol and marijuana are related to pyospermia in infertile men. *J. Urol.* **1990**, *144*, 900–903. [CrossRef]
88. Dixit, V.P.; Gupta, C.L.; Agrawal, M. Testicular degeneration and necrosis induced by chronic administration of cannabis extract in dogs. *Endokrinologie* **1977**, *69*, 299–305.
89. Lewis, S.E.; Paro, R.; Borriello, L.; Simon, L.; Robinson, L.; Dincer, Z.; Riedel, G.; Battista, N.; Maccarrone, M. Long-term use of HU210 adversely affects spermatogenesis in rats by modulating the endocannabinoid system. *Int. J. Androl.* **2012**, *35*, 731–740. [CrossRef]
90. López-Cardona, A.P.; Ibarra-Lecue, I.; Laguna-Barraza, R.; Pérez-Cerezales, S.; Urigüen, L.; Agirregoitia, N.; Gutiérrez-Adán, A.; Agirregoitia, E. Effect of chronic THC administration in the reproductive organs of male mice, spermatozoa and in vitro fertilization. *Biochem. Pharmacol.* **2018**, *157*, 294–303. [CrossRef]
91. Rodriguez, M.C.; Sanchez-Yague, J.; Paniagua, R. Effects of cocaine on testicular structure in the rat. *Reprod. Toxicol.* **1992**, *6*, 51–55. [CrossRef]
92. Samplaski, M.K.; Bachir, B.G.; Lo, K.C.; Grober, E.D.; Lau, S.; Jarvi, K.A. Cocaine Use in the Infertile Male Population: A Marker for Conditions Resulting in Subfertility. *Curr. Urol.* **2015**, *8*, 38–42. [CrossRef]
93. Mendelson, J.H.; Sholar, M.B.; Mutschler, N.H.; Jaszyna-Gasior, M.; Goletiani, N.V.; Siegel, A.J.; Mello, N.K. Effects of intravenous cocaine and cigarette smoking on luteinizing hormone, testosterone, and prolactin in men. *J. Pharmacol. Exp. Ther.* **2003**, *307*, 339–348. [CrossRef]
94. Goletiani, N.V.; Mendelson, J.H.; Sholar, M.B.; Siegel, A.J.; Mello, N.K. Opioid and cocaine combined effect on cocaine-induced changes in HPA and HPG axes hormones in men. *Pharmacol. Biochem. Behav.* **2009**, *91*, 526–536. [CrossRef]
95. Wisniewski, A.B.; Brown, T.T.; John, M.; Frankowicz, J.K.; Cofranceso, J., Jr.; Golub, E.T.; Ricketts, E.P.; Dobs, A.S. Hypothalamic-pituitary-gonadal function in men and women using heroin and cocaine, stratified by HIV status. *Gend. Med.* **2007**, *4*, 35–44. [CrossRef]
96. Insel, J.R.; Dhanjal, N. Pituitary infarction resulting from intranasal cocaine abuse. *Endocr. Pract.* **2004**, *10*, 478–482. [CrossRef]
97. De Lange, T.E.; Simsek, S.; Kramer, M.H.; Nanayakkara, P.W. A case of cocaine-induced panhypopituitarism with human neutrophil elastase-specific anti-neutrophil cytoplasmic antibodies. *Eur. J. Endocrinol.* **2009**, *160*, 499–502. [CrossRef]
98. Gordon, L.A.; Mostofsky, D.I.; Gordon, G.G. Changes in testosterone levels in the rat following intraperitoneal cocaine HCl. *Int. J. Neurosci.* **1980**, *11*, 139–141. [CrossRef]
99. George, V.K.; Li, H.; Teloken, C.; Grignon, D.J.; Lawrence, W.D.; Dhabuwala, C.B. Effects of long-term cocaine exposure on spermatogenesis and fertility in peripubertal male rats. *J. Urol.* **1996**, *155*, 327–331. [CrossRef]
100. Mello, N.K.; Mendelson, J.H.; Negus, S.S.; Kelly, M.; Knudson, I.; Roth, M.E. The effects of cocaine on gonadal steroid hormones and LH in male and female rhesus monkeys. *Neuropsychopharmacology* **2004**, *29*, 2024–2034. [CrossRef]
101. Bracken, M.B.; Eskenazi, B.; Sachse, K.; McSharry, J.E.; Hellenbrand, K.; Leo-Summers, L. Association of cocaine use with sperm concentration, motility, and morphology. *Fertil. Steril.* **1990**, *53*, 315–322. [CrossRef]
102. Li, H.; Jiang, Y.; Rajpurkar, A.; Dunbar, J.C.; Dhabuwala, C.B. Cocaine induced apoptosis in rat testes. *J. Urol.* **1999**, *162*, 213–216. [CrossRef]
103. Li, H.; Jiang, Y.; Rajpurkar, A.; Tefilli, M.V.; Dunbar, J.C.; Dhabuwala, C.B. Lipid peroxidation and antioxidant activities in rat testis after chronic cocaine administration. *Urology* **1999**, *54*, 925–928. [CrossRef]
104. Liechti, M. Novel psychoactive substances (designer drugs): Overview and pharmacology of modulators of monoamine signaling. *Swiss Med. Wkly.* **2015**, *145*, w14043. [CrossRef] [PubMed]
105. Green, A.R.; Mechan, A.O.; Elliott, J.M.; O'Shea, E.; Colado, M.I. The pharmacology and clinical pharmacology of 3,4-methylenedioxymethamphetamine (MDMA, "ecstasy"). *Pharmacol. Rev.* **2003**, *55*, 463–508. [CrossRef] [PubMed]

106. Tsai, S.C.; Chiao, Y.C.; Lu, C.C.; Doong, M.L.; Chen, Y.H.; Shih, H.C.; Liaw, C.; Wang, S.W.; Wang, P.S. Inhibition by amphetamine of testosterone secretion through a mechanism involving an increase of cyclic AMP production in rat testes. *Br. J. Pharmacol.* **1996**, *118*, 984–988. [CrossRef]
107. Tsai, S.C.; Chen, J.J.; Chiao, Y.C.; Lu, C.C.; Lin, H.; Yeh, J.Y.; Lo, M.J.; Kau, M.M.; Wang, S.W.; Wang, P.S. The role of cyclic AMP production, calcium channel activation and enzyme activities in the inhibition of testosterone secretion by amphetamine. *Br. J. Pharmacol.* **1997**, *122*, 949–955. [CrossRef]
108. Chen, L.Y.; Huang, Y.L.; Liu, M.Y.; Leu, S.F.; Huang, B.M. Effects of amphetamine on steroidogenesis in MA-10 mouse Leydig tumor cells. *Life Sci.* **2003**, *72*, 1983–1995. [CrossRef]
109. Yamamoto, Y.; Yamamoto, K.; Hayase, T. Effect of methamphetamine on male mice fertility. *J. Obstet. Gynaecol. Res.* **1999**, *25*, 353–358. [CrossRef]
110. Lin, J.F.; Lin, Y.H.; Liao, P.C.; Lin, Y.C.; Tsai, T.F.; Chou, K.Y.; Chen, H.E.; Tsai, S.C.; Hwang, T.I. Induction of testicular damage by daily methamphetamine administration in rats. *Chin. J. Physiol.* **2014**, *57*, 19–30. [CrossRef]
111. Kaewman, P.; Nudmamud-Thanoi, S.; Thanoi, S. GABAergic Alterations in the Rat Testis after Methamphetamine Exposure. *Int. J. Med. Sci.* **2018**, *15*, 1349–1354. [CrossRef] [PubMed]
112. Dickerson, S.M.; Walker, D.M.; Reveron, M.E.; Duvauchelle, C.L.; Gore, A.C. The recreational drug ecstasy disrupts the hypothalamic-pituitary-gonadal reproductive axis in adult male rats. *Neuroendocrinology* **2008**, *88*, 95–102. [CrossRef] [PubMed]
113. Barenys, M.; Macia, N.; Camps, L.; de Lapuente, J.; Gomez-Catalan, J.; Gonzalez-Linares, J.; Borras, M.; Rodamilans, M.; Llobet, J.M. Chronic exposure to MDMA (ecstasy) increases DNA damage in sperm and alters testes histopathology in male rats. *Toxicol. Lett.* **2009**, *191*, 40–46. [CrossRef] [PubMed]
114. Yamamoto, Y.; Yamamoto, K.; Hayase, T.; Abiru, H.; Shiota, K.; Mori, C. Methamphetamine induces apoptosis in seminiferous tubules in male mice testis. *Toxicol. Appl. Pharmacol.* **2002**, *178*, 155–160. [CrossRef]
115. Alavi, S.H.; Taghavi, M.M.; Moallem, S.A. Evaluation of effects of methamphetamine repeated dosing on proliferation and apoptosis of rat germ cells. *Syst. Biol. Reprod. Med.* **2008**, *54*, 85–91. [CrossRef] [PubMed]
116. Nudmamud-Thanoi, S.; Thanoi, S. Methamphetamine induces abnormal sperm morphology, low sperm concentration and apoptosis in the testis of male rats. *Andrologia* **2011**, *43*, 278–282. [CrossRef]
117. Saberi, A.; Sepehri, G.; Safi, Z.; Razavi, B.; Jahandari, F.; Divsalar, K.; Salarkia, E. Effects of Methamphetamine on Testes Histopathology and Spermatogenesis Indices of Adult Male Rats. *Addict. Health* **2017**, *9*, 199–205.
118. Nudmamud-Thanoi, S.; Sueudom, W.; Tangsrisakda, N.; Thanoi, S. Changes of sperm quality and hormone receptors in the rat testis after exposure to methamphetamine. *Drug Chem. Toxicol.* **2016**, *39*, 432–438. [CrossRef]
119. Mobaraki, F.; Seghatoleslam, M.; Fazel, A.; Ebrahimzadeh-Bideskan, A. Effects of MDMA (ecstasy) on apoptosis and heat shock protein (HSP70) expression in adult rat testis. *Toxicol. Mech. Methods* **2018**, *28*, 219–229. [CrossRef] [PubMed]
120. Vuong, C.; Van Uum, S.H.; O'Dell, L.E.; Lutfy, K.; Friedman, T.C. The effects of opioids and opioid analogs on animal and human endocrine systems. *Endocr. Rev.* **2010**, *31*, 98–132. [CrossRef]
121. Hsieh, A.; DiGiorgio, L.; Fakunle, M.; Sadeghi-Nejad, H. Management Strategies in Opioid Abuse and Sexual Dysfunction: A Review of Opioid-Induced Androgen Deficiency. *Sex. Med. Rev.* **2018**, *6*, 618–623. [CrossRef] [PubMed]
122. Cepeda, M.S.; Zhu, V.; Vorsanger, G.; Eichenbaum, G. Effect of Opioids on Testosterone Levels: Cross-Sectional Study using NHANES. *Pain Med.* **2015**, *16*, 2235–2242. [CrossRef]
123. Fronczak, C.M.; Kim, E.D.; Barqawi, A.B. The insults of illicit drug use on male fertility. *J. Androl.* **2012**, *33*, 515–528. [CrossRef]
124. Abs, R.; Verhelst, J.; Maeyaert, J.; Van Buyten, J.P.; Opsomer, F.; Adriaensen, H.; Verlooy, J.; Van Havenbergh, T.; Smet, M.; Van Acker, K. Endocrine consequences of long-term intrathecal administration of opioids. *J. Clin. Endocrinol. Metab.* **2000**, *85*, 2215–2222. [CrossRef] [PubMed]
125. Lafisca, S.; Bolelli, G.; Franceschetti, F.; Danieli, A.; Tagliaro, F.; Marigo, M.; Flamigni, C. Free and bound testosterone in male heroin addicts. In *Receptors and Other Targets for Toxic Substances*; Springer: Berlin/Heidelberg, Germany, 1985; pp. 394–397.
126. Rasheed, A.; Tareen, I.A. Effects of heroin on thyroid function, cortisol and testosterone level in addicts. *Pol. J. Pharmacol.* **1995**, *47*, 441–444. [PubMed]

127. Daniell, H.W. Hypogonadism in men consuming sustained-action oral opioids. *J. Pain* **2002**, *3*, 377–384. [CrossRef] [PubMed]
128. Safarinejad, M.R.; Asgari, S.A.; Farshi, A.; Ghaedi, G.; Kolahi, A.A.; Iravani, S.; Khoshdel, A.R. The effects of opiate consumption on serum reproductive hormone levels, sperm parameters, seminal plasma antioxidant capacity and sperm DNA integrity. *Reprod. Toxicol.* **2013**, *36*, 18–23. [CrossRef] [PubMed]
129. Bliesener, N.; Albrecht, S.; Schwager, A.; Weckbecker, K.; Lichtermann, D.; Klingmüller, D. Plasma testosterone and sexual function in men receiving buprenorphine maintenance for opioid dependence. *J. Clin. Endocrinol. Metab.* **2005**, *90*, 203–206. [CrossRef]
130. Hallinan, R.; Byrne, A.; Agho, K.; McMahon, C.G.; Tynan, P.; Attia, J. Hypogonadism in men receiving methadone and buprenorphine maintenance treatment. *Int. J. Androl.* **2009**, *32*, 131–139. [CrossRef] [PubMed]
131. Yee, A.; Loh, H.S.; Danaee, M.; Riahi, S.; Ng, C.G.; Sulaiman, A.H. Plasma Testosterone and Sexual Function in Southeast Asian Men Receiving Methadone and Buprenorphine Maintenance Treatment. *J. Sex. Med.* **2018**, *15*, 159–166. [CrossRef] [PubMed]
132. Bawor, M.; Bami, H.; Dennis, B.B.; Plater, C.; Worster, A.; Varenbut, M.; Daiter, J.; Marsh, D.C.; Steiner, M.; Anglin, R.; et al. Testosterone suppression in opioid users: A systematic review and meta-analysis. *Drug Alcohol Depend.* **2015**, *149*, 1–9. [CrossRef]
133. Rubinstein, A.L.; Carpenter, D.M.; Minkoff, J.R. Hypogonadism in men with chronic pain linked to the use of long-acting rather than short-acting opioids. *Clin. J. Pain* **2013**, *29*, 840–845. [CrossRef]
134. Li, S.; Pelletier, G. Opioid regulation of gonadotropin-releasing hormone gene expression in the male rat brain as studied by in situ hybridization. *Neuroreport* **1993**, *4*, 331–333. [CrossRef] [PubMed]
135. Singh, H.H.; Purohit, V.; Ahluwalia, B.S. Methadone blocks dopamine-mediated release of gonadotropins in rat hypothalamus. *Neuroendocrinology* **1982**, *34*, 347–352. [CrossRef]
136. Adams, M.L.; Sewing, B.; Forman, J.B.; Meyer, E.R.; Cicero, T.J. Opioid-induced suppression of rat testicular function. *J. Pharmacol. Exp. Ther.* **1993**, *266*, 323–328. [PubMed]
137. Abdellatief, R.B.; Elgamal, D.A.; Mohamed, E.E. Effects of chronic tramadol administration on testicular tissue in rats: An experimental study. *Andrologia* **2015**, *47*, 674–679. [CrossRef] [PubMed]
138. Ahmadnia, H.; Akhavan Rezayat, A.; Hoseyni, M.; Sharifi, N.; Khajedalooee, M.; Akhavan Rezayat, A. Short-Period Influence of Chronic Morphine Exposure on Serum Levels of Sexual Hormones and Spermatogenesis in Rats. *Nephro-Urol. Mon.* **2016**, *8*, e38052. [CrossRef]
139. Agirregoitia, E.; Valdivia, A.; Carracedo, A.; Casis, L.; Gil, J.; Subiran, N.; Ochoa, C.; Irazusta, J. Expression and localization of delta-, kappa-, and mu-opioid receptors in human spermatozoa and implications for sperm motility. *J. Clin. Endocrinol. Metab.* **2006**, *91*, 4969–4975. [CrossRef]
140. Ibrahim, M.A.; Salah-Eldin, A.E. Chronic Addiction to Tramadol and Withdrawal Effect on the Spermatogenesis and Testicular Tissues in Adult Male Albino Rats. *Pharmacology* **2019**, *103*, 202–211. [CrossRef]
141. Cicero, T.J.; Davis, L.A.; LaRegina, M.C.; Meyer, E.R.; Schlegel, M.S. Chronic opiate exposure in the male rat adversely affects fertility. *Pharmacol. Biochem. Behav.* **2002**, *72*, 157–163. [CrossRef]
142. Sagoe, D.; Molde, H.; Andreassen, C.S.; Torsheim, T.; Pallesen, S. The global epidemiology of anabolic-androgenic steroid use: A meta-analysis and meta-regression analysis. *Ann. Epidemiol.* **2014**, *24*, 383–398. [CrossRef]
143. La Vignera, S.; Condorelli, R.A.; Cannarella, R.; Duca, Y.; Calogero, A.E. Sport, doping and female fertility. *Reprod. Biol. Endocrinol.* **2018**, *16*, 108. [CrossRef] [PubMed]
144. Coward, R.M.; Rajanahally, S.; Kovac, J.R.; Smith, R.P.; Pastuszak, A.W.; Lipshultz, L.I. Anabolic steroid induced hypogonadism in young men. *J. Urol.* **2013**, *190*, 2200–2205. [CrossRef] [PubMed]
145. Christou, M.A.; Christou, P.A.; Markozannes, G.; Tsatsoulis, A.; Mastorakos, G.; Tigas, S. Effects of Anabolic Androgenic Steroids on the Reproductive System of Athletes and Recreational Users: A Systematic Review and Meta-Analysis. *Sports Med.* **2017**, *47*, 1869–1883. [CrossRef] [PubMed]
146. Kanayama, G.; Hudson, J.I.; Pope, H.G., Jr. Illicit anabolic-androgenic steroid use. *Horm. Behav.* **2010**, *58*, 111–121. [CrossRef]
147. Gårevik, N.; Strahm, E.; Garle, M.; Lundmark, J.; Ståhle, L.; Ekström, L.; Rane, A. Long term perturbation of endocrine parameters and cholesterol metabolism after discontinued abuse of anabolic androgenic steroids. *J. Steroid Biochem. Mol. Biol.* **2011**, *127*, 295–300. [CrossRef]

148. Rasmussen, J.J.; Selmer, C.; Østergren, P.B.; Pedersen, K.B.; Schou, M.; Gustafsson, F.; Faber, J.; Juul, A.; Kistorp, C. Former Abusers of Anabolic Androgenic Steroids Exhibit Decreased Testosterone Levels and Hypogonadal Symptoms Years after Cessation: A Case-Control Study. *PLoS ONE* **2016**, *11*, e0161208. [CrossRef]
149. Feinberg, M.J.; Lumia, A.R.; McGinnis, M.Y. The effect of anabolic-androgenic steroids on sexual behavior and reproductive tissues in male rats. *Physiol. Behav.* **1997**, *62*, 23–30. [CrossRef]
150. De Souza, G.L.; Hallak, J. Anabolic steroids and male infertility: A comprehensive review. *BJU Int.* **2011**, *108*, 1860–1865. [CrossRef]
151. Shokri, S.; Aitken, R.J.; Abdolvahhabi, M.; Abolhasani, F.; Ghasemi, F.M.; Kashani, I.; Ejtemaeimehr, S.; Ahmadian, S.; Minaei, B.; Naraghi, M.A.; et al. Exercise and supraphysiological dose of nandrolone decanoate increase apoptosis in spermatogenic cells. *Basic Clin. Pharmacol. Toxicol.* **2010**, *106*, 324–330. [CrossRef] [PubMed]
152. Knuth, U.A.; Maniera, H.; Nieschlag, E. Anabolic steroids and semen parameters in bodybuilders. *Fertil. Steril.* **1989**, *52*, 1041–1047. [CrossRef]
153. Torres-Calleja, J.; González-Unzaga, M.; DeCelis-Carrillo, R.; Calzada-Sánchez, L.; Pedrón, N. Effect of androgenic anabolic steroids on sperm quality and serum hormone levels in adult male bodybuilders. *Life Sci.* **2001**, *68*, 1769–1774. [CrossRef]
154. Liu, P.Y.; Swerdloff, R.S.; Christenson, P.D.; Handelsman, D.J.; Wang, C.; Hormonal Male Contraception Summit Group. Rate, extent, and modifiers of spermatogenic recovery after hormonal male contraception: An integrated analysis. *Lancet* **2006**, *367*, 1412–1420. [CrossRef]
155. Nieschlag, E.; Vorona, E. MECHANISMS IN ENDOCRINOLOGY: Medical consequences of doping with anabolic androgenic steroids: Effects on reproductive functions. *Eur. J. Endocrinol.* **2015**, *173*, R47–R58. [CrossRef] [PubMed]

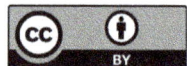

© 2019 by the authors. Licensee MDPI, Basel, Switzerland. This article is an open access article distributed under the terms and conditions of the Creative Commons Attribution (CC BY) license (http://creativecommons.org/licenses/by/4.0/).

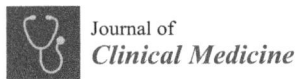

Article

Testicular Function of Childhood Cancer Survivors: Who Is Worse?

Ylenia Duca [1], Andrea Di Cataldo [2], Giovanna Russo [2], Emanuela Cannata [2], Giovanni Burgio [1], Michele Compagnone [1], Angela Alamo [1], Rosita A. Condorelli [1], Sandro La Vignera [1,*] and Aldo E. Calogero [1]

1. Andrology and Endocrinology Unit, Department of Clinical and Experimental Medicine, University of Catania, 95123 Catania, Italy; ylenia.duca@gmail.com (Y.D.); burgio.giovanni88@libero.it (G.B.); michele.compagnone22@tiscali.it (M.C.); angela.alamo1986@gmail.com (A.A.); rosita.condorelli@unict.it (R.A.C.); acaloger@unict.it (A.E.C.)
2. Pediatric Oncohematology Unit, Department of Clinical and Experimental Medicine, University of Catania, 95123 Catania, Italy; adicata@unict.it (A.D.C.); diberuss@unict.it (G.R.); e.cannata80@gmail.com (E.C.)
* Correspondence: sandrolavignera@unict.it; Tel.: +39-095-378-1435

Received: 16 November 2019; Accepted: 11 December 2019; Published: 13 December 2019

Abstract: Background: A multi-disciplinary approach has led to an improvement in prognosis of childhood cancers. However, in parallel with the increase in survival rate, there is a greater occurrence of long-term toxicity related to antineoplastic treatment. Hypogonadism and infertility are among the most frequent endocrinological sequelae in young adult childhood cancer survivors. The aim of this study was to identify which category of patients, grouped according to diagnosis, therapy, and age at treatment, shows the worst reproductive function in adulthood. Methods: We evaluated morpho-volumetric development of the testis, endocrine function of the hypothalamic–pituitary–gonadal axis, and sperm parameters in 102 young adult childhood cancer survivors. Results: Overall, about one-third of patients showed low total testicular volume, total testosterone (TT) <3.5 ng/mL, and altered sperm count. Hodgkin's disease, hematopoietic stem cell transplantation, and non-cranial irradiation associated to chemotherapy were risk factors for poor gonadal function. Patients treated in pubertal age showed lower total testicular volume; however, the difference was due to more gonadotoxic treatment performed in older age. Testicular volume was more predictive of spermatogenesis than follicle-stimulating hormone (FSH), while anti-Müllerian hormone (AMH) was not useful in the evaluation of testicular function of male childhood cancer survivors. Conclusions: Pre-pubertal subjects at high risk of future infertility should be candidates for testicular tissue cryopreservation.

Keywords: childhood cancer survivors; infertility; hypogonadism; testicular volume; azoospermia; chemotherapy; radiotherapy; stem cell transplantation; lymphoma; leukemia

1. Introduction

Cancer in childhood and adolescence represents a rare pathology; however, it has a great biological interest and an extreme social and public health importance. A multi-disciplinary approach has led to an evident improvement in prognosis and quality of life for these patients who, more and more frequently, reach adulthood. Indeed, the drafting of increasingly effective diagnostic-therapeutic protocols has allowed to increase the 5-year survival rate from the 58% recorded at the end of the 1980s to around the 80% [1]. Therefore, in parallel with the increase in number of children and adolescents who reach adulthood after having undergone treatment for cancer, there is a greater occurrence of long-term toxicities related to therapies carried out in pediatric age.

Endocrine disorders are highly prevalent among cancer survivors; it has been estimated that 40–50% of survivors will develop at least one endocrinopathy over the course of their lifetime [2]. Among the negative endocrine long-term effects of antineoplastic treatments, gonadal failure and subsequent subfertility/infertility is one of the most frequent and most important for its economic and psycho-social implications.

The gonadotoxic potential of some treatments, such as alkylating agents and testicular irradiation, is well known [3]. Chemotherapy-induced testicular damage is drug-specific and dose-related: the extent of the damage and the speed of recovery depend on the agent used and the dose received. Similarly, radiotherapy damages testicular germinal cells in a dose-dependent manner. However, not all children who undergo the same antineoplastic treatments will become infertile because individual susceptibility plays an important role in conditioning reproductive outcomes. Since adult testicular function is unpredictable, all boys already capable of ejaculating should, as a precaution, cryopreserve sperm before undergoing antineoplastic treatments. Pre-pubertal patients who do not yet have spermarche represent the category with major concerns about fertility, because the cryopreservation of testicular tissue with subsequently auto-graft is still an experimental procedure performed by few centers and with low probability of success [3].

Another issue regards the age at treatment. In past decades, it has been reported that patients treated at pre-pubertal age were protected from chemotherapy-induced testicular damage [4,5]. Authors hypothesized that the protective effect of very-young age was due to the relative quiescence of the germinal epithelium in the early stages of life [4,5]. Other research questioned this assumption [6–9], but recent studies are lacking.

In this study, we evaluated the endocrine function of the hypothalamic-pituitary-gonadal axis, the morpho-volumetric development of the testis, and sperm production in young adult men who underwent chemotherapy, irradiation, and/or bone marrow transplantation for the treatment of childhood cancer. The aim was to identify which, among these treatments, has the worst effect on testicular function in adulthood, for establishing which categories of childhood cancer patients should be recommended for testicular tissue cryopreservation. We also evaluated the influence of diagnosis and age at treatment on future fertility.

2. Materials and Methods

2.1. Study Population

This study involved 102 male long-term survivors of childhood cancer who underwent annual outpatient visits at the Pediatric Oncohematology Unit of the University Hospital "G. Rodolico" in Catania, Italy, between March 2018 and July 2019.

We enrolled patients aged between 16 and 40 years at the time of the visit, who had been treated with chemotherapy only, chemotherapy plus radiotherapy, and/or bone marrow transplantation and who were declared disease-free for at least 5 years. Patients treated with surgery only, testicular irradiation or orchiectomy for testicular neoplasia, and/or who were in testosterone replacement therapy at the time of the visit were excluded.

Each patient underwent a thorough health assessment including medical history collection, general and andrological physical examination, and scrotal ultrasound. Most patients underwent blood sampling for the dosage of luteinizing hormone (LH), follicle-stimulating hormone (FSH), and total testosterone (TT). A part of the patients underwent also anti-Müllerian hormone (AMH) dosage. Patients who accepted to undergo sperm analysis provided a semen sample.

2.2. Scrotal Ultrasound

All patients underwent testicular ultrasound, performed by the medical staff of the Andrology and Endocrinology Unit of the University Hospital "Gaspare Rodolico" (Catania, Italy).

By ultrasound, we evaluated testicular volume, echotexture, and echo structure. Total testicular volume, resulting from the sum of the volume of the two testes, was considered normal when ≥24 mL. Echo structure and texture were considered normal if they were normoechoic and homogeneous.

By ecocolor Doppler, performed in basal conditions and during the Valsalva maneuver, it was also possible to explore the presence of varicocele and to assess its grading according to the Sarteschi classification. Varicocele was considered clinically significant in presence of basal, uni- or bilateral, venous reflux (grade IV Sarteschi).

Ultrasound scrotal evaluation was performed through an Esaote Mylab25 ultrasound scanner with a 7.5 MHz linear probe.

2.3. Hormone Essays

The measurement of LH, FSH, and TT was performed on blood samples by electrochemiluminescence (ECLIA). AMH was evaluated by one-step simultaneous enzyme immunoassay ("sandwich").

Blood was collected at the same time as the oncohematological outpatient visit, that may occur in the morning or in the afternoon. For this reason, fasting was not required.

2.4. Semen Analysis

Patients were asked to deliver a semen sample by masturbation after a sexual abstinence of 3–5 days. The collection was carried out in a dedicated room adjacent to the seminology laboratory of the Andrology and Endocrinology Unit, within a sterile, wide-mouthed plastic container. The samples were analyzed by a qualified medical operator soon after liquefaction and, in any case, within an hour after ejaculation. The semen analysis was performed in accordance with the 2010 World Health Organization manual (5th edition) [10].

Semen samples with no visible sperm were centrifuged at 3000× g for 10 min. If no sperms were found after examination of 40 microscopic fields of the sediment at 400× magnification, the sample was considered azoospermic.

2.5. Statistical Analysis

The data obtained were analyzed with PHStat and RealStatistics add-on for Excel and all results were expressed as mean ± SD. The Shapiro–Wilk test was used to establish the normality of the distribution. Data with normal distribution was compared with Student's t-test; while non-parametric data was examined with the Mann–Whitney U test. Pearson's correlation coefficient was used to assess correlations between sperm concentration, testicular volume, and FSH. Simple and multivariate regression was performed for testicular volume. One-tailed $p \leq 0.05$ was considered significant.

2.6. Ethical Approval

The protocol was approved by the internal Institutional Review Board (ethical approval code: 27/2018), and informed consent was obtained from each participant after full explanation of the purpose and nature of all procedures used. The study was conducted in accordance with the principles expressed in the Declaration of Helsinki.

All patients were made aware of the results of their clinical tests and who showed hormonal, ultrasound, and/or seminal alterations was included in a clinical and instrumental monitoring program at the Andrology and Endocrinology Unit of the University Hospital of Catania.

3. Results

One hundred and fifty-six male patients visited the outpatient clinic dedicated to long-term survivors of childhood cancer between March 2018 and July 2019. Among them, 54 patients were excluded: 41 were too young, 2 were too old, 3 had finished antineoplastic treatment less than five years before, 1 was treated with surgery alone, 6 underwent unilateral orchiectomy for testicular tumor, 1 was on testosterone replacement therapy for an already diagnosed primary hypogonadism (Figure 1).

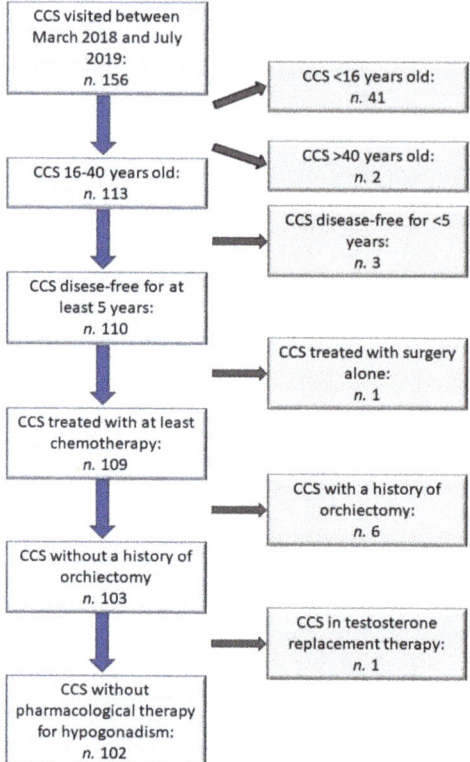

Figure 1. Flow-chart of sample selection process. CCS: Childhood cancer survivors.

A total of 102 patients, aged 16–38 years, were enrolled. Mean age at diagnosis was 6.2 ± 4.2 years; mean age at enrollment was 23.2 ± 5.4 years (Table 1). Main diagnoses were acute lymphoblastic leukemia (ALL) (*n*. 67), non-Hodgkin's lymphoma (NHL) (*n*. 11), Hodgkin's disease (HD) (*n*. 8), Wilms tumor (WT) (*n*. 5), acute myeloid leukemia (AML) (*n*. 4), and hepatoblastoma (HB) (*n*. 3). The other 4 patients had been affected by histiocytosis, nasopharyngeal carcinoma, rhabdomyosarcoma, and Ewing's sarcoma (Figure 2). All patients had been treated with at least chemotherapy, according to the protocols of Italian Association of Pediatric Hematology and Oncology (AIEOP), based on the type and stage of the malignancy. In addition to chemotherapy, 28 patients also received irradiation and 5 underwent hematopoietic stem cell transplantation (SCT).

Table 1. Clinical features of childhood cancer survivors, overall and according to therapy and age at the time of treatment (mean ± DS). AMH: anti-Müllerian hormone: CCS: childhood cancer; CO: chemotherapy only; CRc: chemotherapy plus cranial irradiation; CRn: chemotherapy plus non-cranial irradiation; FSH: follicle-stimulating hormone; LH: luteinizing hormone; STC: stem cell transplantation; TT: total testosterone; TV: testicular volume. Reference values: TV ≥ 24 mL, LH 1.14–8.75 UI/L, FSH 0.95–11.95 UI/L, TT ≥3.5 ng/mL (gray zone 2.3–3.5 ng/mL), AMH 0.73–16.05 ng/mL, sperm concentration >39 × 10^6/mL.

Clinical Features	All CSS	CO	CRc	CRn	STC	<10 Years	≥10 Years
Age at diagnosis (years)	6.2 ± 4.2	5.7 ± 3.8	6.5 ± 5.1	8.2 ± 4.2	6.6 ± 5.2	4.2 ± 2.3	12.3 ± 2.0
Age at enrollment (years)	23.2 ± 5.4	22.1 ± 4.7	26.9 ± 5.6	22.4 ± 5.2	27.0 ± 5.7	22.9 ± 5.6	24.0 ± 4.7
Total TV (mL)	26.6 ± 8.9	29.4 ± 6.7	27.6 ± 6.9	18.1 ± 9.2	7.9 ± 4.5	27.5 ± 8.5	24.0 ± 9.8
LH (UI/L)	4.1 ± 2.3	3.6 ± 1.7	3.2 ± 2.1	5.2 ± 2.8	8.6 ± 2.9	4.0 ± 2.0	4.5 ± 3.1
FSH (UI/L)	5.5 ± 5.9	3.4 ± 2.0	4.1 ± 2.6	11.7 ± 8.4	17.5 ± 10.2	4.6 ± 3.9	7.8 ± 9.2
TT (ng/mL)	4.5 ± 1.8	4.6 ± 1.9	5.4 ± 1.2	3.8 ± 1.2	3.2 ± 0.9	4.5 ± 1.8	4.5 ± 1.9
AMH (ng/mL)	5.7 ± 5.0	6.2 ± 6.3	/	3.9 ± 2.2	8.1 ± 2.3	6.5 ± 5.8	4.0 ± 1.3
Sperm concentration (10^6/mL)	46.8 ± 45.3	52.0 ± 46.1	64.1 ± 46.3	12.5 ± 25.0	0 ± 0	48.2 ± 48.1	43.8 ± 40.8

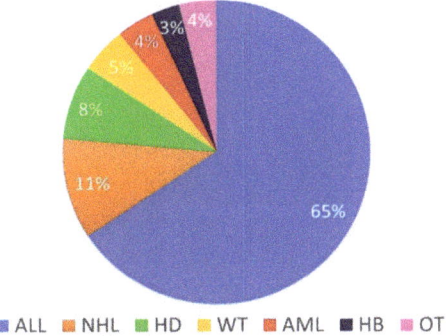

Figure 2. Frequency of diagnosis in 102 childhood cancer survivors. ALL: acute lymphoblastic leukemia; AML: acute myeloid leukemia; HB: hepatoblastoma; HD: Hodgkin's disease; NHL: non-Hodgkin lymphoma; OT: other malignancies (histiocytosis, nasopharyngeal carcinoma, rhabdomyosarcoma, and Ewing's sarcoma); WT: Wilms tumor.

3.1. Grouping According to Diagnosis, Therapy, and Age of Treatment

Childhood cancer survivors were allocated to five categories according to diagnosis: ALL, NHL, HD, WT, and others (OT). The OT group included all diagnosis which occurred in less than 5 patients (acute myeloid leukemia, hepatoblastoma, histiocytosis, nasopharyngeal carcinoma, rhabdomyosarcoma, and Ewing's sarcoma).

Patients were also classified according to the treatment received: chemotherapy only (CO), chemotherapy plus radiotherapy (CR), hematopoietic stem cell transplantation (SCT). The CR group was further divided into two subgroups: chemotherapy plus cranial irradiation (CRc) and chemotherapy plus non-cranial irradiation (CRn).

According to the age of treatment, patients were subdivided into two group: patients treated in prepubertal age (<10 years old) and patients treated in pubertal age (≥10 years old). The cut-off of 10 years was chosen based on the report of Nielsen and colleagues indicating the age of 11.7 years as the lower range of the interval at which spermarche occurs. Thus, under the age of 10, all subjects were probably pre-pubertal [11]. The same cut-off was previously used in other studies [12,13].

3.2. Testicular Morpho-Volumetry

All enrolled childhood cancer survivors underwent scrotal ultrasound. Mean right, left, and total testicular volume were in the normal range (Table 1). However, total testicular volume was low (<24 mL) in one third of patients (n. 38). Twenty out of 102 patients (19.6%) had a clinically significant varicocele (≥IV grade of Sarteschi classification).

After patients' grouping according to diagnosis, only the HD group showed significantly lower total testicular volume values compared to the overall sample of childhood cancer survivors ($p < 0.001$) (Table 2, Figure 3).

Table 2. Clinical features of childhood cancer survivors according to diagnosis (mean ± DS). ALL: acute lymphoblastic leukemia; AMH: anti-Müllerian hormone; FSH: follicle-stimulating hormone; HD: Hodgkin's disease; LH: luteinizing hormone; NHL: non-Hodgkin's lymphoma; TT: total testosterone; TV: testicular volume; OT: other malignancies; WT: Wilms tumor. Reference values: TV ≥24 mL, LH 1.14–8.75 UI/L, FSH 0.95–11.95 UI/L, TT ≥3.5 ng/mL (gray zone 2.3–3.5 ng/mL), AMH 0.73–16.05 ng/mL, sperm concentration >39 × 10^6/mL.

Clinical Features	ALL	NHL	HD	WT	OT
Age at diagnosis (years)	5.7 ± 3.9	6.8 ± 3.3	10.3 ± 4.1	2.4 ± 1.9	7.2 ± 4.9
Age at enrollment (years)	23.6 ± 5.7	22.3 ± 4.5	24.1 ± 5.4	22.4 ± 6.3	21.9 ± 5
Total TV (mL)	28.1 ± 8.1	23.8 ± 10	12.5 ± 3.5	28.8 ± 8.8	27 ± 9.5
LH (UI/L)	3.9 ± 2	4.2 ± 3.5	6.6 ± 2.8	4.2 ± 2.7	3.9 ± 2.5
FSH (UI/L)	4.1 ± 3.1	6.7 ± 7.1	15.8 ± 8.8	8 ± 9.4	6.2 ± 8.6
TT (ng/mL)	4.9 ± 1.9	3.7 ± 1.4	3.3 ± 0.7	5.2 ± 1	4.1 ± 1.2
AMH (ng/mL)	5.2 ± 2.6	23.2	5.4	2.3	2.9
Sperm concentration (10^6/mL)	47.2 ± 36.5	52 ± 46.1	0 ± 0	/	68.8 ± 94.4

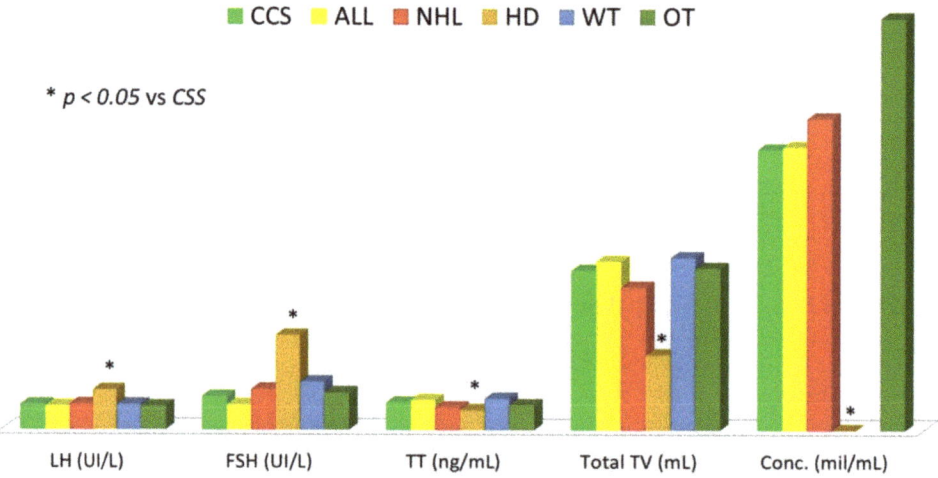

Figure 3. Comparison of hormonal values, total testicular volume, and sperm concentration among childhood cancer survivors grouped according to diagnosis. ALL: acute lymphoblastic leukemia; CCS: childhood cancer survivors; Conc.: sperm concentration; FSH: follicle-stimulating hormone; HD: Hodgkin's disease; LH: luteinizing hormone; NHL: non-Hodgkin lymphoma; TT: total testosterone; TV: testicular volume; OT: other malignancies; WT: Wilms tumor.

After grouping according to therapy, the CO group showed significantly higher total testicular volume compared to overall sample of childhood cancer survivors ($p = 0.015$); the CR group had significantly lower total testicular volume than the CO group ($p < 0.001$); the SCT group showed significantly lower total testicular volume than both CO ($p < 0.001$) and CR groups ($p = 0.001$). After further subdividing patients belonging to the CR group in two different categories according to the irradiated site (cranial or non-cranial), total testicular volume of CRc patients showed no statistically significant differences compared to the CO group. On the contrary, the CRn group had significantly lower total testicular volume compared to both CO ($p < 0.001$) and CRc ($p = 0.002$) groups (Table 1, Figure 4).

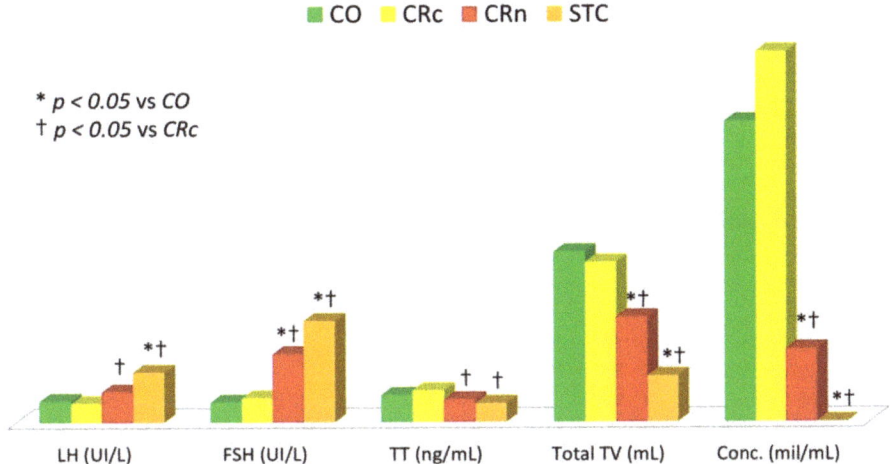

Figure 4. Comparison of hormonal values, total testicular volume, and sperm concentration among childhood cancer survivors grouped according to therapy. CO: chemotherapy only; Conc.: sperm concentration; CRc: chemotherapy plus cranial irradiation; CRn: chemotherapy plus non-cranial irradiation; FSH: follicle-stimulating hormone; LH: luteinizing hormone; STC: stem cell transplantation; TT: total testosterone; TV: testicular volume.

After subdivision for age of treatment, patients treated when they were ≥10 years old showed slightly but significantly lower total testicular volume compared to patient aged <10 years at the time of treatment ($p = 0.046$) (Table 1). However, data became not significant when adjusted for diagnosis and treatment. In patients treated with chemotherapy only (CO), there was a trend for a lower testicular volume in survivors treated in pubertal age, but the difference did not reach statistical significance ($p = 0.052$). To confirm our assumption, we built a multivariate regression model, including age at the time of treatment, diagnosis, modality of treatment, and presence of varicocele. With backward procedure, we were able to establish that therapy was the only variable significantly related to testicular volume, alone explaining 36% of the volume variability.

3.3. Endocrine Function of the Hypothalamic–Pituitary–Testis Axis

Eighty-seven childhood cancers survivors underwent hormonal evaluation. Overall mean hormonal values were in the normal range (Table 1). Three out of 87 patients (3.4%) and 5/87 patients (5.7%) exhibited respectively below or above normal LH levels. None of the patients had reduced FSH values, while 8/87 patients (9.2%) showed FSH levels above normal range. Twenty eight of the 84 patients (33.3%) had testosterone values <3.5 ng/mL; however, only 5 patients (6%) showed frankly reduced TT levels (<2.3 ng/mL). Testosterone values of three patients were missing because of lab errors.

Of blood samples from 17 patients, we also evaluated AMH concentrations. None of the childhood cancers survivors had low AMH levels, while only 1 patient had AMH values above normal.

After patients' grouping according to diagnosis, only the HD group showed significantly higher LH and FSH values and significantly lower TT values compared to overall sample of childhood cancer survivors ($p = 0.013$, <0.001, and 0.027, respectively) (Table 2, Figure 3).

After grouping according to therapy, the CO group showed slightly but significantly lower FSH values compared to the overall sample of childhood cancer survivors ($p = 0.047$); the CR group had significantly higher FSH values than the CO group ($p = 0.009$); the SCT group showed significantly higher FSH and LH values compared to both CO ($p = 0.001$ and $p < 0.001$) and CR groups ($p = 0.004$ and $p = 0.008$). After further subdividing the CR group patients in two different categories according to the irradiated site (cranial or non-cranial), the CRc group showed hormonal values comparable to the CO group, except for TT values that were slightly but significantly higher ($p = 0.042$). On the contrary, the CRn group had significantly higher FSH levels than both CO ($p < 0.001$) and CRc ($p = 0.001$) groups, and higher LH and lower TT values than the CRc group ($p = 0.02$ and 0.003, respectively) (Table 1, Figure 4).

After subdivision for age of treatment, the two groups (<10 years old and ≥10 years old) showed no significant differences in hormone levels (Table 1).

3.4. Sperm Parameters

Thirty-four patients accepted to undergo sperm analysis. Overall mean sperm concentration and count were in the normal range (Table 1). Sperm count was reduced in 7/34 patients (20.6%), while azoospermia was found in 6/34 patients (17.7%). Overall, 38.2% of patients showed low or absent sperm production. All azoospermic patients had primary testicular disease, characterized by FSH levels >8 UI/L and low testicular volume, and had undergone radiotherapy or SCT. Among oligozoospermic patients, 5 had normal FSH values and testicular volume and 2 had normal FSH values and slightly reduced testicular volume. Four of them showed clinically significant varicocele.

After patients' grouping according to diagnosis, only the HD group showed significantly lower sperm concentration compared to the overall sample of childhood cancer survivors ($p = 0.029$) (Table 2, Figure 3).

After grouping according to therapy, only the SCT group showed reduced sperm concentration compared to the CO group ($p = 0.004$) and to the overall sample of childhood cancer survivors ($p = 0.025$). When the CR group was further subdivided into two categories according to the irradiated site, the CRn group showed lower sperm concentration than both CO and CRc groups ($p = 0.007$ and 0.036, respectively) (Table 1, Figure 4).

After subdivision for age of treatment, there was no significant difference between the two groups (<10 years old and ≥10 years old) in terms of sperm concentration (Table 1).

Pearson's correlation coefficient revealed that sperm concentration was related more to testicular volume ($\rho = 0.51$, $p = 0.002$) than FSH ($\rho = -0.43$, $p = 0.01$).

4. Discussion

Only one third of patients accepted to undergo sperm analysis. Many childhood cancer survivors refused saying they did not want to know anything about their reproductive function or that they were not willing to have children, now or in the future. The same reluctance was described by other authors [12,14,15]. This common attitude among childhood cancer survivors has led authors to look for surrogate markers of spermatogenesis to be used in infertility screening. Inhibin B has proved to be a better marker for spermatogenesis than FSH [12,14]. However, in some studies, testicular size was shown to be a predictor of sperm production even better than serum inhibin B [16]. The difference in the predictive power of testicular volume depends on the applied measurement methods. Most of the studies that did not show statistically significant differences between testicular volume of patients and controls used the orchidometer [12]. To our knowledge, ours is one of the few studies about childhood cancer survivors in which testicular volume has been measured by ultrasound. This is a strength, since it has been shown that orchidometer is less accurate than ultrasound in volume evaluation, especially in testes smaller than 18 mL [17]. By ultrasound, we showed that testicular volume is a predictor of poor spermatogenesis better than FSH, but we were not able to compare it with inhibin B since we could not measure this hormone. AMH showed no usefulness in gonadal evaluation of young adult male long-term childhood cancer survivors. The only patient with elevated AMH levels was 22 years old and he was treated for NHL at 3 years of age with chemotherapy only. He exhibited normal gonadotropin levels, TT levels in the "grey zone", and modestly decreased total testicular volume, but he refused to undergo sperm analysis.

In this study we found a high percentage of patients (one third) with suboptimal TT levels; however, a low prevalence of overt hypogonadism (TT ≤2.3 ng/mL) and altered LH levels were recorded. This probably occurred because blood samples for hormone essays were not drawn in standardized condition. According to Endocrine Society guidelines, testosterone must be measured in the morning after 8 h of fasting and the diagnosis must be confirmed repeating the blood sampling a second time under the same conditions [18]. We were unable to follow these indications because, to improve patients' compliance, we performed blood sampling at the same time of the outpatient visit, which sometimes took place also in the afternoon.

In the past decades, it has been hypothesized that pre-pubertal testis is less sensitive than post-pubertal testis to chemotherapy-induced damage. Some reports supported this assumption [4,5], while other studies did not [6–9]. The Childhood Cancer Survivor Study reported that only boys <4 years of age at diagnosis were more likely to sire a pregnancy later in life than those who were 15–20 years of age at diagnosis [19]. In our study, the only parameter marginally related to the age at diagnosis was testicular volume, but a more careful analysis found that the difference was due to therapy: in pubertal and post-pubertal age, HD diagnosis and combined therapy with alkylating drugs and irradiation were more frequent, while in early childhood LLA and WT were the most common diagnosis, requiring less gonadotoxic therapy.

Data from the Childhood Cancer Survivor Study showed that the main risk factors for male infertility after antineoplastic treatment were: diagnosis of HD, testicular irradiation with ≥7.5 Gy, and alkylating agent dose score ≥2; while pituitary irradiation was not related to impaired fertility [19]. Our study confirmed that cranial irradiation with up to 24 Gy does not affect pituitary gonadotropin secretion as shown by the fact that childhood cancer survivors who underwent chemotherapy and cranial irradiation showed similar hormone levels than patients treated with only chemotherapy. None of our patients received cranial radiation dose >24 Gy.

Unfortunately, we have not been able to subdivide patients according to alkylating agent dose score because for many of them (especially the older ones), it was not possible to trace the exact dose of chemotherapy received. Thus, we preferred to divide patients according to the diagnosis, assuming that patients suffering from the same pathology had received similar treatment schemes and could represent a homogeneous group.

Similar to the results of the Childhood Cancer Survivor Study, we found that HD was the diagnosis with the worst testicular function. HD patients usually undergo higher doses of alkylating and alkylating-like agents; however, they routinely also undergo thoracic and/or abdominal irradiation. It is known that not only direct testicular irradiation but also scattered dose could be responsible for testicular damage [20]. We hypothesize that testicular damage in HD patients could be partially due to scattered testicular irradiation. Our assumption is supported by the finding that childhood cancers survivors who underwent non-cranial irradiation have poorer testicular function than both patients who underwent chemotherapy only and chemotherapy plus cranial irradiation, independently from diagnosis. Indeed, the CRn group also included patients who underwent non-cranial irradiation for other malignancies than HD (nasopharyngeal carcinoma, rhabdomyosarcoma, Wilms tumor, Ewing's sarcoma).

As expected, patients who underwent HSCT had poor testicular function: all of them had low testicular volume and all of them except one had high FSH levels. Among them, the two patients who accepted to perform semen analysis were azoospermic.

Currently, fertility preservation treatments for pre-pubertal patients who do not yet produce mature spermatozoa are lacking. Some centers have started to cryopreserve immature testicular tissue from pre-pubertal boys before starting chemotherapy treatment. In 2015, seven centers in Europe had already collected and stored more than 260 pre-pubertal testicular tissue samples, with biopsies undertaken only when treatment was deemed at high risk for later fertility complications [3]. It is not yet certain if such cryopreserved tissue can be successfully used later to restore fertility in humans. However, the generation of sperm-like cells after 3D culture of isolated spermatogonial cells obtained from testis biopsies taken from pre-pubertal boys undergoing chemotherapy treatment has been recently described [21]. In a murine model, complete spermatogenesis was achieved through the in vitro culture of spermatogonial germ cells; the obtained mature spermatozoa have then been used to produce viable embryos through in vitro fertilization/ intracytoplasmic sperm injection (IVF/ICSI) [22]. Another frontier of fertility preservation in male childhood cancer survivors is the transplantation of spermatogonial stem cells or frozen-thawed immature testicular tissue grafted back into the adult. This technique has been successful in producing functional gametes in animal models, including non-human primates and mice, and healthy offspring have been produced through IVF/ICSI using sperm derived from xenografted immature testicular tissue. The concerns are about the possible reintroduction of malignant cells in case of unapparent leukemic infiltration of the xenografted tissue [3].

Instead of trying to restore fertility, an alternative strategy would be the development of interventions aimed at preventing chemotherapy- or radiation-induced testicular damage. Cytoprotective agents that specifically protect the pre-pubertal testis without interfering with the toxicity to cancer cells could potentially be employed as part of the treatment regimen. In vivo animal studies investigated the effects of the administration of antioxidants (amifostine, carnitine, ginseng intestinal metabolite I, vitamin C, and curcumin) prior to chemotherapy reporting contrasting results [3].

In post pubertal boys and men, a prophylactic down-regulation of the pituitary gland by gonadotropin-releasing hormone (GnRH) agonists or testosterone to induce a quiescent state in the gonads was proposed. This approach was attempted for the belief that the prepubescent testis was less sensitive to gonadal toxicity than the active adult one, as demonstrated by old studies [5]. However, more recent data—including ours—showed that both pre-pubertal and post-pubertal testis are sensible to the gonadotoxic damage of chemo- and radiotherapy [23].

Regarding radioprotection techniques, modern shielding systems allow to reduce the scattered radiation to the testis up to 1% of the prescribed dose. However, the received dose depends primarily on the distance from the field edge to the gonads [24]. Modifications in irradiation techniques has reduced radiation dose scattered to testis during treatment of pelvic fields. For example, proton radiotherapy significantly reduced scattered dose to normal tissues compared with intensity-modulated radiotherapy in male patients treated for pediatric pelvic rhabdomyosarcoma [25]. This could suggest a wider use of proton radiotherapy instead of intensity-modulated radiotherapy also in other pediatric malignancies in order to better safeguard future reproductive function; however, further studies are needed.

5. Conclusions

Our study showed that patients with the worst reproductive function among childhood cancers survivors are those with previous diagnosis of HD and treated with non-cranial irradiation in addition to chemotherapy and/or STC. Patients treated with chemotherapy only and chemotherapy plus cranial irradiation did not show, as a group, any impairment of testicular function. Age at diagnosis (pre-pubertal or pubertal) does not also seem to influence gonadal function of childhood cancer survivors in young adulthood. However, generalizations cannot always be applied to the specific case.

Indeed, due to individual susceptibility to chemotherapy- and radiotherapy-induced testicular damage, the resumption of spermatogenesis after different kinds of treatments tends to be unpredictable, and studies on spermatogenesis in long-term cancer survivors have shown evidence of persistent azoospermia or severe oligozoospermia in up to 24% of patients [13,26]. For these reasons, sperm cryopreservation—if possible—is always indicated before starting antineoplastic treatment. In 20% of Tanner II boys, spermiogenesis has already started, allowing cryopreservation of sperm from that age. Thus, pubertal boys with testicular volumes greater than 10–12 mL should give semen samples before undergoing antineoplastic therapy [20].

Finally, our study showed that testicular volume evaluated by ultrasound is more predictive of spermatogenesis than FSH. Our preliminary data also indicate that AMH is not useful in the evaluation of testicular function in childhood cancer survivors.

Author Contributions: Y.D. performed scrotal ultrasound, carried out the analysis and interpretation of data, and drafted the article. A.D.C. and G.R. conceived the study. A.E.C. and S.L.V. designed the study and revised critically the article. E.C. was responsible for the enrollment of patients. A.A. performed sperm analysis. G.B. and M.C. performed scrotal ultrasound. R.A.C. participated in data acquisition, analysis and interpretation of data. All authors read and approved the final manuscript.

Funding: This study was funded by the 2016/2018 Research Plan of University of Catania, Department of Clinical and Experimental Medicine (project #B: "Evaluation of long-term harmful effects of chemotherapy and radiotherapy on various organs in childhood cancer survivors").

Acknowledgments: We thank the medical students Samuele Paxhia and Evelina Moliteo for their contribution to data collection and reporting.

Conflicts of Interest: The authors declare no conflict of interest. The funders had no role in the design of the study; in the collection, analyses, or interpretation of data; in the writing of the manuscript, or in the decision to publish the results.

References

1. Miller, K.D.; Siegel, R.L.; Lin, C.C.; Mariotto, A.B.; Kramer, J.L.; Rowland, J.H.; Stein, K.D.; Alteri, R.; Jemal, A. Cancer treatment and survivorship statistics, 2016. *CA Cancer J. Clin.* **2016**, *66*, 271–289. [CrossRef] [PubMed]
2. Sklar, C.A.; Antal, Z.; Chemaitilly, W.; Cohen, L.E.; Follin, C.; Meacham, L.R.; Murad, M.H. Hypothalamic-Pituitary and Growth Disorders in Survivors of Childhood Cancer: An Endocrine Society Clinical Practice Guideline. *J. Clin. Endocrinol. Metab.* **2018**, *103*, 2761–2784. [CrossRef] [PubMed]
3. Allen, C.M.; Lopes, F.; Mitchell, R.; Spears, N. How does chemotherapy treatment damage the prepubertal testis? *Reproduction* **2018**. [CrossRef] [PubMed]
4. Sherins, R.J.; Olweny, C.L.; Ziegler, J.L. Gynecomastia and gonadal dysfunction in adolescent boys treated with combination chemotherapy for Hodgkin's disease. *N. Engl. J. Med.* **1978**, *299*, 12–16. [CrossRef] [PubMed]
5. Rivkees, S.A.; Crawford, J.D. The relationship of gonadal activity and chemotherapy-induced gonadal damage. *JAMA* **1988**, *259*, 2123–2125. [CrossRef]
6. Green, D.M.; Brecher, M.L.; Lindsay, A.N.; Yakar, D.; Voorhess, M.L.; MacGillivray, M.H.; Freeman, A.I. Gonadal function in pediatric patients following treatment for Hodgkin disease. *Med. Pediatr. Oncol.* **1981**, *9*, 235–244. [CrossRef]
7. Jaffe, N.; Sullivan, M.P.; Ried, H.; Boren, H.; Marshall, R.; Meistrich, M.; Maor, M.; da Cunha, M. Male reproductive function in long-term survivors of childhood cancer. *Med. Pediatr. Oncol.* **1988**, *16*, 241–247. [CrossRef]
8. Aubier, F.; Flamant, F.; Brauner, R.; Caillaud, J.M.; Chaussain, J.M.; Lemerle, J. Male gonadal function after chemotherapy for solid tumors in childhood. *J. Clin. Oncol.* **1989**, *7*, 304–309. [CrossRef]
9. Kenney, L.B.; Laufer, M.R.; Grant, F.D.; Grier, H.; Diller, L. High risk of infertility and long term gonadal damage in males treated with high dose cyclophosphamide for sarcoma during childhood. *Cancer* **2001**, *91*, 613–621. [CrossRef]
10. World Health Organization, Department of Reproductive Health and Research. *WHO Laboratory Manual for the Examination and Processing of Human Semen*, 5th ed.; World Health Organization: Geneva, Switzerland, 2010.
11. Nielsen, C.T.; Skakkebaek, N.E.; Richardson, D.W.; Darling, J.A.; Hunter, W.M.; Jørgensen, M.; Nielsen, A.; Ingerslev, O.; Keiding, N.; Müller, J. Onset of the release of spermatozoa (spermarche) in boys in relation to age, testicular growth, pubic hair, and height. *J. Clin. Endocrinol. Metab.* **1986**, *62*, 532–535. [CrossRef]

12. van Casteren, N.J.; van der Linden, G.H.; Hakvoort-Cammel, F.G.; Hählen, K.; Dohle, G.R.; van den Heuvel-Eibrink, M.M. Effect of childhood cancer treatment on fertility markers in adult male long-term survivors. *Pediatr. Blood Cancer* **2009**, *52*, 108–112. [CrossRef] [PubMed]
13. Romerius, P.; Ståhl, O.; Moëll, C.; Relander, T.; Cavallin-Ståhl, E.; Wiebe, T.; Giwercman, Y.L.; Giwercman, A. High risk of azoospermia in men treated for childhood cancer. *Int. J. Androl.* **2011**, *34*, 69–76. [CrossRef] [PubMed]
14. van Beek, R.D.; Smit, M.; van den Heuvel-Eibrink, M.M.; de Jong, F.H.; Hakvoort-Cammel, F.G.; van den Bos, C.; van den Berg, H.; Weber, R.F.; Pieters, R.; de Muinck Keizer-Schrama, S.M. Inhibin B is superior to FSH as a serum marker for spermatogenesis in men treated for Hodgkin's lymphoma with chemotherapy during childhood. *Hum. Reprod.* **2007**, *22*, 3215–3222. [CrossRef] [PubMed]
15. Lähteenmäki, P.M.; Arola, M.; Suominen, J.; Salmi, T.T.; Andersson, A.M.; Toppari, J. Male reproductive health after childhood cancer. *Acta Paediatr.* **2008**, *97*, 935–942. [CrossRef]
16. Jahnukainen, K.; Heikkinen, R.; Henriksson, M.; Cooper, T.G.; Puukko-Viertomies, L.R.; Mäkitie, O. Semen quality and fertility in adult long-term survivors of childhood acute lymphoblastic leukemia. *Fertil. Steril.* **2011**, *96*, 837–842. [CrossRef]
17. Lin, C.C.; Huang, W.J.; Chen, K.K. Measurement of testicular volume in smaller testes: How accurate is the conventional orchidometer? *J. Androl.* **2009**, *30*, 685–689. [CrossRef]
18. Bhasin, S.; Brito, J.P.; Cunningham, G.R.; Hayes, F.J.; Hodis, H.N.; Matsumoto, A.M.; Snyder, P.J.; Swerdloff, R.S.; Wu, F.C.; Yialamas, M.A. Testosterone Therapy in Men with Hypogonadism: An Endocrine Society Clinical Practice Guideline. *J. Clin. Endocrinol. Metab.* **2018**, *103*, 1715–1744. [CrossRef]
19. Green, D.M.; Kawashima, T.; Stovall, M.; Leisenring, W.; Sklar, C.A.; Mertens, A.C.; Donaldson, S.S.; Byrne, J.; Robison, L.L. Fertility of male survivors of childhood cancer: A report from the Childhood Cancer Survivor Study. *J. Clin. Oncol.* **2010**, *28*, 332–339. [CrossRef]
20. Vakalopoulos, I.; Dimou, P.; Anagnostou, I.; Zeginiadou, T. Impact of cancer and cancer treatment on male fertility. *Hormones (Athens)* **2015**, *14*, 579–589. [CrossRef]
21. Abofoul-Azab, M.; AbuMadighem, A.; Lunenfeld, E.; Kapelushnik, J.; Shi, Q.; Pinkas, H.; Huleihel, M. Development of Postmeiotic Cells in vitro from Spermatogonial Cells of Prepubertal Cancer Patients. *Stem. Cells Dev.* **2018**, *27*, 1007–1020. [CrossRef]
22. Sato, T.; Katagiri, K.; Yokonishi, T.; Kubota, Y.; Inoue, K.; Ogonuki, N.; Matoba, S.; Ogura, A.; Ogawa, T. In vitro production of fertile sperm from murine spermatogonial stem cell lines. *Nat. Commun.* **2011**, *2*, 472. [CrossRef] [PubMed]
23. Lee, S.H.; Shin, C.H. Reduced male fertility in childhood cancer survivors. *Ann. Pediatr. Endocrinol. Metab.* **2013**, *18*, 168–172. [CrossRef] [PubMed]
24. Fraass, B.A.; Kinsella, T.J.; Harrington, F.S.; Glatstein, E. Peripheral dose to the testes: The design and clinical use of a practical and effective gonadal shield. *Int. J. Radiat. Oncol. Biol. Phys.* **1985**, *11*, 609–615. [CrossRef]
25. Cotter, S.E.; Herrup, D.A.; Friedmann, A.; Macdonald, S.M.; Pieretti, R.V.; Robinson, G.; Adams, J.; Tarbell, N.J.; Yock, T.I. Proton radiotherapy for pediatric bladder/prostate rhabdomyosarcoma: Clinical outcomes and dosimetry compared to intensity-modulated radiation therapy. *Int. J. Radiat. Oncol. Biol. Phys.* **2011**, *81*, 1367–1373. [CrossRef] [PubMed]
26. López Andreu, J.A.; Fernández, P.J.; Ferrís i Tortajada, J.; Navarro, I.; Rodríguez-Ineba, A.; Antonio, P.; Muro, M.D.; Romeu, A. Persistent altered spermatogenesis in long-term childhood cancer survivors. *Pediatr. Hematol. Oncol.* **2000**, *17*, 21–30. [CrossRef]

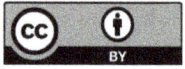

© 2019 by the authors. Licensee MDPI, Basel, Switzerland. This article is an open access article distributed under the terms and conditions of the Creative Commons Attribution (CC BY) license (http://creativecommons.org/licenses/by/4.0/).

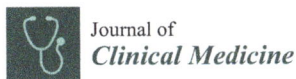

Article

Thyroid Hormones and Spermatozoa: In Vitro Effects on Sperm Mitochondria, Viability and DNA Integrity

Rosita A. Condorelli, Sandro La Vignera *, Laura M. Mongioì, Angela Alamo, Filippo Giacone, Rossella Cannarella and Aldo E. Calogero

Department of Clinical and Experimental Medicine, University of Catania, Via S. Sofia 78, 95123 Catania, Italy; rosita.condorelli@unict.it (R.A.C.); lauramongioi@hotmail.it (L.M.M.); angela.alamo1986@gmail.com (A.A.); filippogiacone@yahoo.it (F.G.); roxcannarella@gmail.com (R.C.); acaloger@unict.it (A.E.C.)
* Correspondence: sandrolavignera@unict.it; Tel.: +39-0953781435 or +39-0953781180

Received: 1 May 2019; Accepted: 23 May 2019; Published: 27 May 2019

Abstract: The aim of this study wasto assess the in vitro effects of levothyroxine (LT4) on conventional and bio-functional sperm parameters and its implications on fertility. Patients with male idiopathic infertility were enrolled and subjected to examination of the seminal fluid and capacitation according to the WHO 2010 criteria and flow cytometric sperm analysis for the evaluation of bio-functional sperm parameters. LT4 significantly increased the percentage of spermatozoa with high mitochondrial membrane potential (MMP), decreased the percentage of spermatozoa with low MMP and increased sperm motility already at a concentration of 0.9 pmol L^{-1}. Therefore, LT4 significantly reduced sperm necrosis and lipid peroxidation ameliorating chromatin compactness. These effects of LT4 were evident at a concentration of 2.9 pmol L^{-1}, close to the physiological free-thyroxine (FT4) concentrations in the seminal fluid of euthyroid subjects. We showed a beneficial role of thyroid hormones on sperm mitochondrial function, oxidative stress and DNA integrity. The results of this in vitro study could have a clinical application in patients with idiopathic infertility, clarifying the role of thyroid function on male fertility.

Keywords: thyroid hormones; spermatozoa; sperm parameters; sperm mitochondrial potential; sperm motility

1. Introduction

It is known that the thyroid hormones (THs), 3,5,3′-triiodothyronine (T_3) and thyroxine (T_4) impact the reproductive function, and thyroid dysfunction is associated with an adverse effect on fertility, both in men [1,2] and women [3]. Indeed, hyperthyroidism or thyrotoxicosis damages spermatogenesis causing maturation arrest, impairs mitochondrial activity and alters the antioxidant systems in rats [4]. Hyperthyroidism results in asthenozoospermia in humans [5–7]. In rats, hypothyroidism shows sperm abnormalities partly similar to those reported in hyperthyroidism with an arrest of spermatogenesis, reduction of sperm vitality and an increase of oxidative stress with lipid peroxidation [4,8,9], as well as asthenozoospermia in humans [7]. These semen alterations are reversible both in hypo- and hyperthyroidism and disappear upon achieving euthyroidism [7].

However, the role of THs on male reproductive function and on sperm parameters is still unclear and the scientific evidence is conflicting. To date, all in vitro studies have been performed on animal models; no study has addressed bio-functional and conventional sperm parameters regarding humans.

The presence of thyroid hormone receptors (TR) in rat [10] and human [11] testes suggests a possible role for TH. Moreover, TR are expressed in the whole testis as well as in Sertoli, Leydig and germ cells, epididymis and penis [12].

Thyroid hormones can act with a direct effect on sperm cells as well as on Sertoli and Leydig cells. Moreover, THs act by genomic and nongenomic effects [13].

Genomic effects derive from the binding of T3 with its TR in the nucleus of Sertoli and Leydig cells: it activates gene transcription and protein synthesis, regulating their proliferation and differentiation. T_3 regulates steroidogenesis through TRα1 in Leydig cells, but Sertoli cells are the main target of T_3 action in the testes [14].

Nongenomic effects result from the binding of THs with nonnuclear TR in cytoplasmatic membrane, cytoplasm, cytoskeleton and mitochondria where sperm motility is regulated by cAMP pathways.

Some evidences suggest a negative impact of T_4 on male fertility by showing that it impairs human sperm motility acting with a TR-dependent mechanism [15], decreases the number of spermatozoa/spermatids in the seminiferous tubular lumen and alters the seminal vesicles in animal models [16]. Moreover, T_3 and T_4 could damage DNA by increasing reactive oxygen species production [17]. Conversely, other evidences show that free T_4 concentration seems inversely correlated with sperm DNA damage with a potential protective effect [18] and the treatment with levothyroxine (LT4) increases the weights of both epididymis and testis [19].

The aim of the study was to evaluate whether THs were able to improve the sperm quality (apoptosis, chromatin/DNA integrity and mitochondrial function), to ameliorate oxidative stress, sperm motility and recovery after capacitation.

To accomplish this, the effect of levothyroxine (LT4) on conventional and bio-functional sperm parameters and their implications on fertility were evaluated in vitro.

2. Materials and Methods

2.1. Patient Selection

The study was conducted in vitro on 15 euthyroid men (mean age 31.2 ± 6.4 years) with idiopathic infertility.

2.2. Sperm Analysis and Preparation

Sperm analysis was conducted according to the World Health Organization criteria 2010 [20]. Subsequently, spermatozoa were aliquoted and incubated at 37 °C under 5% CO_2 with increasing concentrations of LT4 (Sigma-Aldrich S.r.l. Milan, Italy) (0, 0.9, 2.9, 9.9 pmol L^{-1}) for 30 min to evaluate the effects on:

- Sperm progressive motility.
- Sperm recovery after capacitation by swim-up technique using the Biggers, Whitten, and Whittingham medium (BWW) with capacitating properties. Spermatozoa were then recovered from the supernatant according to their capacity to migrate from the bottom of the test tube to the surface.
- Bio-functional sperm parameters by flow cytometry: Mitochondrial membrane potential (MMP), vitality, early apoptosis, late apoptosis, necrosis, chromatin compactness, DNA fragmentation and lipid peroxidation (LP).

To date, no study investigated the free-thyroxine FT4 concentration in the semen of men. The LT4 doses used in this study were selected on the basis of the concentrations of FT4 previously tested in the semen of unselected euthyroid men similar to those found in enrolled patients (mean: 3.15 ± 0.7 pmol L^{-1}) by chemoluminescence. Moreover, we chose a time of 30 min to reduce the time-dependent sperm damage (reduction of motility, apoptosis, etc.) also considering the analysis times of the seminal fluid, swim-up, etc.

2.3. Flow Cytometric Analysis

Flow cytometric analysis was performed using flow cytometer CytoFLEX (Beckman Coulter Life Science, Milan, Italy). The CytoFLEX was equipped with two solid state lasers and six total fluorescence channels (four 488 nm and two 638 nm). We used the FL1 detectors for the green (525 nm), FL2 for the orange (575 nm) and FL3 for the red (620 nm) fluorescence; 100,000 events (low velocity) were measured for each sample. The debris was gated out, by drawing a region on forward versus side scatter dot plot enclosing the population of cells of interest. Computed compensation was made before performing all the analyses. Data were analyzed by the software CytExpert 1.2.

2.4. Evaluation of Sperm Apoptosis/Vitality

The externalization of phosphatidylserine (PS) on the outer cell surface is used as an indicator of early apoptosis. The assessment of PS externalization was performed using annexin V, a protein that binds selectively the PS in presence of calcium ions. Therefore, marking simultaneously the cells with annexin V and propidium iodide (PI), we distinguished: Alive (with intact cytoplasmic membrane), apoptotic or necrotic spermatozoa. Staining with annexin V and PI was obtained using a commercially available kit (Annexin V-FITC Apoptosis, Beckman Coulter, IL, Milan, Italy). An aliquot containing 0.5×10^6 mL^{-1} was suspended in 0.5 mL of buffer containing 10 µL of annexin V-FITC and 20 µL of PI and incubated for 10 min in the dark. After incubation, the sample was analyzed by the fluorescence channels 525/40 BP (FITC) and 585/42 BP, 610/20 BP, 690/50 BP (PI). The different pattern of staining allowed us to identify the different cell populations: FITC negative and PI negative indicate alive sperm cells, FITC positive and PI negative indicate spermatozoa in early apoptosis and FITC positive and PI positive indicate sperm cells in late apoptosis.

2.5. Evaluation of the Mitochondrial Membrane Potential

The evaluation of MMP was performed using the lipophilic probe 5,5',6,6'-tetrachloro-1,1',3,3'tetraethyl-benzimidazolylcarbocyanine iodide (JC-1) which is able to selectively penetrate into mitochondria when it is in monomeric form, emitting at 527 nm. Therefore, JC-1 excitated at 490 nm is able to form aggregates emitting at 590 nm in relation to the membrane potential. When the mitochondrial membrane becomes more polarized, the fluorescence changes reversibly from green to orange. In cells with normal membrane potential, JC-1 is in the mitochondrial membrane in form of aggregates emitting in an orange fluorescence, while in the cells with low membrane potential it remains in the cytoplasm in a monomeric form, emitting a green fluorescence. As regards the sample preparation, we incubated an aliquot containing 1×10^6 mL^{-1} spermatozoa with JC-1 (JC-1 Dye, Mitochondrial Membrane Potential Probe, Labochem Science, Catania, Italy) for 10 min, at a temperature of 37 °C and in the dark; after incubation, the cells were washed in PBS and analyzed (FL1 and FL3) obtaining two different populations:

- spermatozoa with high mitochondrial membrane potential (H-MMP)
- spermatozoa with low mitochondrial membrane potential (L-MMP).

2.6. Assessment of DNA Fragmentation

The evaluation of DNA fragmentation was performed by the TUNEL assay. This method uses terminal deoxynucleotidyl transferase (TdT), an enzyme that polymerizes at the level of DNA breaks, modifying nucleotides conjugated to a fluorochrome. The TUNEL assay was performed using a commercially available kit (Apoptosis Mebstain kit, DBA s.r.l, Milan, Italy). To obtain a negative control, TdT was omitted from the reaction mixture; the positive control was obtained by pre-treating spermatozoa (about 0.5×10^6) with 1 mg/ml of deoxyribonuclease I, not containing RNAse, at 37 °C for 60 min prior to staining. After fixation (4% paraformaldehyde) and permeabilization of the plasma membrane (ethanol 70%), we incubated an aliquot containing 0.5–1×10^6 mL^{-1} spermatozoa for 60 min, at a temperature of 37 °C; after incubation, the cells were washed in PBS and analyzed (FL1).

2.7. Degree of Chromatin Compactness Assessment

Chromatin compactness assessment was evaluated after a process of cell membrane permeabilization; in this way fluorophore was able to penetrate the nucleus. An aliquot of 1×10^6

spermatozoa was incubated with LPR DNA-Prep Reagent containing 0.1% potassium cyanate, 0.1% NaN3, non-ionic detergents, saline and stabilizers (Beckman Coulter, IL, Milan, Italy) in the dark at room temperature for 10 min. It was then incubated with Stain DNA-Prep Reagent containing 50 µgm L^{-1} of PI (<0.5%), RNase A (4 KUnitz/mL), <0.1% NaN3, saline and stabilizers (Beckman Coulter, IL) in the dark at room temperature for 30 min. The cells were analyzed (FL3).

2.8. Sperm Membrane Lipid Peroxidation Evaluation

LP evaluation was performed using the probe BODIPY (581/591) C11 (Invitrogen, Thermo Fisher Scientific, Eugene, Oregon, USA), which responds to the attack of free oxygen radicals changing its emission spectrum from red to green after being incorporated into cell membranes. This change of the emission is detected by the flow cytometer which provides an estimate of the degree of peroxidation. About 2×10^6 of spermatozoa were incubated with 5 mM of the probe for 30 min in a final volume of 1 mL. After washing with PBS, flow cytometric analysis was conducted using the 525/40 BP (FITC) and 585/42 BP (PE) fluorescence channels.

This study was approved by the Ethics Committee of University teaching Hospital of Policlinico-Vittorio Emanuele, University of Catania (Catania, Italy).

All methods were performed in accordance with the relevant guidelines and regulations. All participants were asked for and provided their informed consent.

2.9. Statistical Analysis

The results are expressed as mean±SEM throughout the study. Statistical analysis of the data was performed using Student's t-test, when possible, and by one-way analysis of variance (ANOVA) followed by the Duncan's Multiple Range test. SPSS 22.0 for Windows was used for statistical analysis (SPSS Inc., Chicago, USA). Results with a p-value less than 0.05 were accepted as statistically significant.

3. Results

The conventional sperm parameters (mean ± SEM) of enrolled men are shown in Table 1. We reported also the seminal FT4 measurement of the same patients in Table 1.

Table 1. Conventional sperm parameters, FT4 seminal measurements, anthropometric parameters and hormone measurements in serum (mean ± SEM) of enrolled men.

	Patients (n = 15)
Concentration (10^6 mL^{-1})	42.80 ± 12.0
Total count (10^6 ejaculate^{-1})	107.00 ± 30
Progressive motility (%)	39.80 ± 3.3
Total motility (%)	77.90 ± 9.8
Normal form (%)	8.30 ± 0.8
Leukocytes (10^6 mL^{-1})	0.70 ± 0.2
Seminal FT4 (pmol L^{-1})	3.15 ± 0.7
Age	31.2 ± 6.4
BMI (kg m^{-2})	24.2 ± 1.3
Waist circumference (cm)	94.0 ± 2.4
TSH (µUI m L^{-1})	2.1 ± 0.5
FT4 (pmol L^{-1})	10.2 ± 0.9
FT3 (pmol L^{-1})	4.7 ± 0.8
FSH (UI L^{-1})	2.3 ± 0.1
LH (UI L^{-1})	2.4 ± 0.2
Total testosterone (ng mL^{-1})	6.1 ± 1.1

Effects on sperm motility: LT4 significantly increased (10%) sperm progressive motility at a concentration of 0.9 pmol L^{-1} compared to LT4 0, whereas LT4 decreased (9% and 10% respectively) sperm motility at concentrations of 2.9 and 9.9 pmol L^{-1} ($p < 0.05$ vs. LT4 0) (Figure 1).

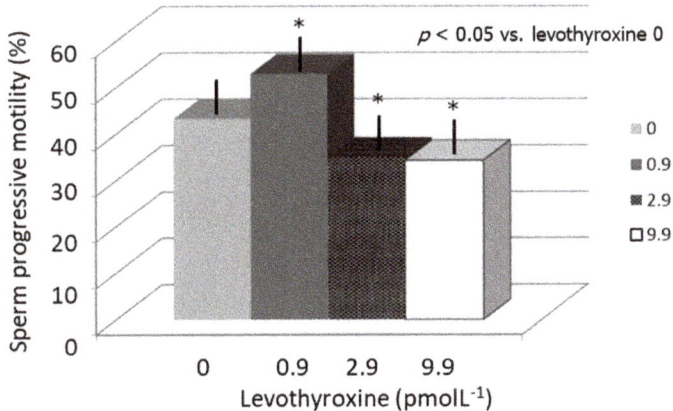

Figure 1. Sperm progressive motility after incubation with increasing concentrations of levothyroxine (LT4).

Effects on bio-functional sperm parameters: LT4 significantly increased the percentage of spermatozoa with high MMP and decreased the percentage of spermatozoa with low MMP. This effect was similar for all the three concentration of LT4 tested ($p < 0.05$ vs. LT4 0) (Figure 2). Moreover, LT4 reduced the percentage of spermatozoa in necrosis at the concentration of 2.9 and 9.9 pmol L^{-1} ($p < 0.05$ vs. LT4 0) while chromatin compactness already improved to a concentration of 0.9 and became statistically significant at the concentration of 9.9 pmol L^{-1} (Figure 3). Finally, LP improved already at a concentration of 0.9 pmol L^{-1} ($p < 0.05$ vs. LT4 0) (Figure 3). DNA fragmentation did not vary for all the three concentration of LT4 tested. Non-significant data are shown in Table 2.

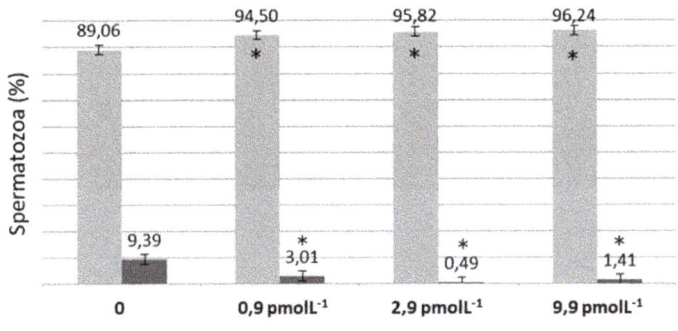

Figure 2. Percentage of spermatozoa with high (H-MMP) and low (L-MMP) membrane mitochondrial potential after incubation with increasing concentrations of levothyroxine (LT4).

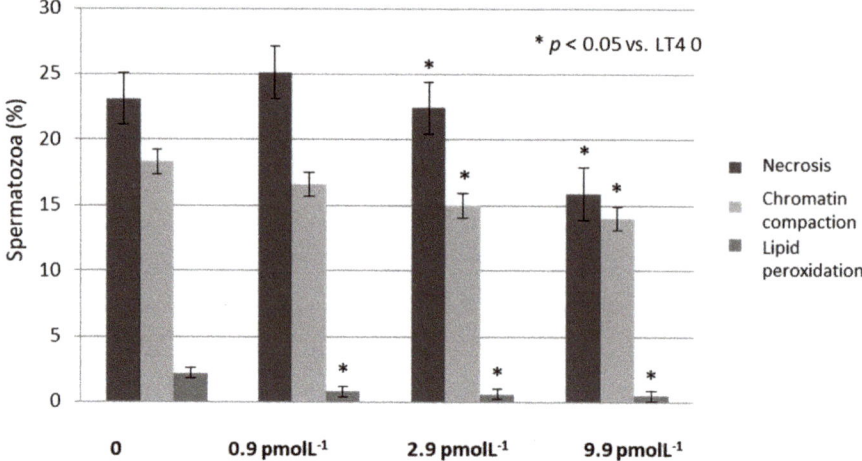

Figure 3. Sperm necrosis, chromatin compactness and lipid peroxidation after incubation with increasing concentrations of levothyroxine (LT4).

Effects on sperm recovery: The number of spermatozoa recovered by capacitation did not change significantly after incubation with LT4 though it increased at a concentration of 0.9 pmol L^{-1} compared to LT4 0 (Table 2).

Table 2. Bio-functional sperm parameters and sperm recovery after incubation with increasing concentrations of levothyroxine (LT4).

Sperm Parameters	LT4 Concentrations			
	0	0.9 pmol L^{-1}	2.9 pmol L^{-1}	9.9 pmol L^{-1}
Alive	65.2 ± 4.6	53.6 ± 8.8	57.3 ± 6.2	54.0 ± 9.3
Early Apoptosis	2.0 ± 0.8	1.5 ± 0.5	1.6 ± 0.7	1.8 ± 0.5
Late apoptosis	18.6 ± 8.6	19.9 ± 8.8	15.2 ± 6.4	23.9 ± 7.8
DNA fragmentation	3.4 ± 0.5	3.8 ± 0.6	4.1 ± 0.7	3.9 ± 0.7
Sperm recovery by swim-up	18.7 ± 8.8	21.3 ± 10.0	14.9 ± 7.7	11.9 ± 10.8

The anthropometric parameters and hormone measurements in serum (mean ± SEM) of enrolled patients are shown in Table 1.

4. Discussion

Many aspects of the possible role of THs are yet to be clarified. Our study investigated the in vitro effects of LT4 on human sperm motility and bio-functional sperm parameters at physiological concentrations as measured in the seminal fluid, for the first time. Accordingly, we selected a physiological dose (2.9 pmol L^{-1}) of LT4 and concentrations respectively lower (0.9 pmol L^{-1}) and higher (9.9 pmol L^{-1}) for our in vitro experiments.

We hypothesized a relationship between sperm motility and mitochondrial function as previously described [21–23]. Our results showed that MMP improved significantly after incubation with LT4 already at a concentration of 0.9 pmol L^{-1}. Similarly, LT4 was able to increase sperm motility at the same concentration, but at higher concentrations than 0.9 pmol L^{-1}, sperm progressive motility decreased significantly. These data confirmed the relationship between these two spermatic parameters, so we hypothesized that LT4 improving MMP also stimulated sperm motility until substrates are exhausted with a subsequent decline in motility itself.

Xian and colleagues showed a negative impact of LT4 on human sperm motility at a concentration of 10 μM [15]. These findings confirm our results, allowing us to understand that high concentrations, which simulate an in vitro condition of hyperthyroidism, damage spermatozoa.

Moreover, the decreased sperm motility observed with the two highest concentrations of LT4 used in the present study may be due to an excessive consumption of substrates after exposure to higher concentrations of LT4 (greater than 0.9 pmol L^{-1}). Indeed, LT4 improved MMP by increasing oxidative phosphorylation and sperm motility related to this biochemical mechanism until no further substrates were available. A condition of hyperthyroidism alters cytochrome c oxidase activity decreasing mitochondrial activity [4]. In addition, the number of spermatozoa recovered by swim-up increased only at the concentration of 0.9 pmol L^{-1}, and did not improve at higher concentrations due to the concomitant reduction in sperm motility. Based on our findings, we hypothesize that slight additions of LT4, in a seminal fluid with constant concentrations of LT4 as in euthyroid men, may result in improved sperm motility. If the concentration of LT4 exceeds this level, these parameters worsen as in a clinical situation of hyperthyroidism due to excessive consumption of the substrates.

Therefore, we showed a beneficial effect of LT4 on sperm oxidative stress that ameliorates after incubation with 0.9 pmol L^{-1}. This effect may explain the reduction in the percentage of spermatozoa in necrosis or with altered chromatin compactness after incubation with LT4.

The in vitro effects of LT4 on viability, chromatin compactness and LP can be explained by the presence of the nuclear TR in spermatozoa [14]. Dobrzynska et al., suggested that T_3 and T_4 could damage DNA by increasing reactive oxygen species production at the concentration of 80 μM [17] but these concentrations are more elevated compared to the physiological doses found in the seminal fluid. Conversely, a condition of hypothyroidism impairs the antioxidant defense system and testicular physiology [9]. We showed that, near physiological concentrations, LT4 improved oxidative stress without altering sperm DNA fragmentation.

Therefore, slight additions of seminal LT4 could be useful for improving the semen sample so that it could be used for assisted reproductive techniques.

5. Conclusion

We showed a role of THs on sperm mitochondrial function. In addition, LT4 seems to act by decreasing the oxidative stress and improving DNA integrity. Therefore, we could achieve a beneficial effect on both conventional and bio-functional sperm parameters maintaining thyroid hormone concentrations sufficient and mostly constant in the seminal fluid. The clinical application of these data could be useful in some cases of idiopathic infertility. Further studies should be undertaken to better investigate the intracellular and biomolecular mechanisms supporting these findings. The next step on this topic could be to investigate hypothyroid infertile and euthyroid fertile men to better understand the role of thyroid hormones on male reproductive function.

Author Contributions: R.A.C. conceived the work and wrote the paper. L.M.M., A.A., F.G., R.C. provided methodological aspects and S.L.V. and A.E.C. revised the paper critically and gave final approval. All authors read and approved the final manuscript.

Funding: This research did not receive any specific grant from any funding agency in the public, commercial or not-for-profit sector.

Conflicts of Interest: On behalf of all authors, the corresponding author states that there is no conflict of interest.

References

1. Wagner, M.S.; Wajner, S.M.; Maia, A.L. Is there a role for thyroid hormone on spermatogenesis? *Microsc. Res. Tech.* **2009**, *72*, 796–808. [CrossRef]
2. La Vignera, S.; Vita, R.; Condorelli, R.A.; Mongioì, L.M.; Presti, S.; Benvenga, S.; Calogero, A.E. Impact of thyroid disease on testicular function. *Endocrine* **2017**, *58*, 397–407. [CrossRef]
3. Dittrich, R.; Beckmann, M.W.; Oppelt, P.G.; Hoffman, I.; Lotz, I.; Kuwert, T.; Mueller, A. Thyroid hormone receptors and reproduction. *J. Reprod. Immunol.* **2011**, *90*, 58–66. [CrossRef]

4. Romano, R.M.; Gomes, S.N.; Cardoso, N.C.; Schiessl, L.; Romano, M.A.; Oliveira, C.A. New insights for male infertility revealed by alterations in spermatic function and differential testicular expression of thyroid-related genes. *Endocrine* **2017**, *55*, 607–617. [CrossRef] [PubMed]
5. Abalovich, M.; Levalle, O.; Hermes, R.; Scaglia, H.; Aranda, C.; Zylbersztein, C.; Oneto, A.; Aquilano, D.; Gutierrez, S. Hypothalamic-pituitary-testicular axis and seminal parameters in hyperthyroid males. *Thyroid* **1999**, *9*, 857–863. [CrossRef]
6. Hudson, R.W.; Edwards, A.L. Testicular function in hyperthyroidism. *J. Androl.* **1992**, *13*, 117–124. [PubMed]
7. Krassas, G.E.; Poppe, K.; Glinoer, D. Thyroid function and human reproductive health. *Endocrine Rev.* **2010**, *31*, 702–755. [CrossRef]
8. Choudhury, S.; Chainy, G.B.; Mishro, M.M. Experimentally induced hypo- and hyper-thyroidism influence on the antioxidant defence system in adult rat testis. *Andrologia* **2003**, *35*, 131–140. [CrossRef] [PubMed]
9. Sahoo, D.K.; Roy, A.; Bhanja, S.; Chainy, G.B. Hypothyroidism impairs antioxidant defence system and testicular physiology during development and maturation. *Gen. Comp. Endocrinol.* **2008**, *156*, 63–70. [CrossRef] [PubMed]
10. Buzzard, J.J.; Morrison, J.R.; O'Bryan, M.K.; Song, Q.; Wreford, N.G. Developmental expression of thyroid hormone receptors in the rat testis. *Biol. Reprod.* **2000**, *62*, 664–669. [CrossRef] [PubMed]
11. Jannini, E.A.; Crescenzi, A.; Rucci, N.; Screponi, E.; Carosa, E.; De Matteis, A.; Macchia, E.; D'Amati, G.; D'Armiento, M. Ontogenetic pattern of thyroid hormone receptor expression in the human testis. *J. Clin. Endocrinol. Metab.* **2000**, *85*, 3453–3457. [CrossRef] [PubMed]
12. Carosa, E.; Lenzi, A.; Jannini, E.A. Thyroid hormone receptors and ligands, tissue distribution and sexual behavior. *Mol. Cell Endocrinol.* **2017**, *30*, 1–11. [CrossRef]
13. La Vignera, S.; Vita, R. Thyroid dysfunction and semen quality. *Int. J. Immunopathol. Pharmacol.* **2018**. [CrossRef]
14. Fumel, B.; Froment, P.; Holzenberger, M.; Livera, G.; Monget, P.; Fouchecourt, S. Expression of domnant-negative thyroid hormone receptor alpha1 in Leydig and Sertoli cells demonstrates no additional defect compared with expression in Sertoli cells only. *PLoS ONE* **2015**, *10*, e01119392. [CrossRef] [PubMed]
15. Xian, H.; Wang, F.; Teng, W.; Yang, D.; Zhang, M. Thyroid hormone induce a p53-dependent DNA damage through PI3K/Akt activation in spem. *Gene* **2017**, *615*, 1–7. [CrossRef]
16. Jacob, T.N.; Pandey, J.P.; Raghuveer, K.; Sreenivasulu, G.; Gupta, A.D.; Yoshikuni, M.; Jagota, A.; Senthilkumaran, B. Thyroxine-induced alterations in the testis and seminal vesicles of air-breathing catfish, Clariasgariepinus. *Fish Physiol. Biochem.* **2005**, *31*, 271–274. [CrossRef]
17. Dobrzynska, M.M.; Baumgartner, A.; Anderson, D. Antioxidant modulate thyroid hormone and noradrenaline induced DNA damage in human sperm. *Mutagenesis* **2004**, *19*, 325–330. [CrossRef] [PubMed]
18. Meeker, J.D.; Singh, N.P.; Hauser, R. Serum concentrations of estradiol and free T4 are inversely correlated with sperm DNA damage in men from an infertility clinic. *J. Androl.* **2008**, *29*, 379–388. [CrossRef] [PubMed]
19. Jiang, J.Y.; Umezu, M.; Sato, E. Characteristics of infertility and the improvement of fertility by thyroxine treatment in adult male hypothyroid rdw rats. *Biol. Reprod.* **2000**, *63*, 1637–1641. [CrossRef]
20. World Health Organization. *WHO Laboratory Manual for the Examination and Processing of Human Semen*, 5th ed.; Cambridge University Press: Cambridge, UK, 2010.
21. Paoli, D.; Gallo, M.; Rizzo, F.; Baldi, E.; Francavilla, S.; Lenzi, A.; Lombardo, F.; Gandini, L. Mitochondrial membrane potential profile and its correlation with increasing sperm motility. *Fertil. Steril.* **2011**, *95*, 2315–2319. [CrossRef] [PubMed]
22. Ferramosca, A.; Provenzano, S.; Coppola, L.; Zara, V. Mitochondrial respiratory efficiency is positively correlated with human sperm motility. *Urology* **2012**, *79*, 809–814. [CrossRef]
23. Moscatelli, N.; Spagnolo, B.; Pisanello, M.; Lemma, E.D.; De Vittorio, M.; Zara, V.; Pisanello, F.; Ferramosca, A. Single-cell-based evaluation of sperm progressive motility via fluorescent assessment of mitochondria membrane potential. *Sci. Rep.* **2017**, *7*, 17931. [CrossRef]

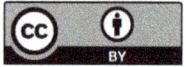

© 2019 by the authors. Licensee MDPI, Basel, Switzerland. This article is an open access article distributed under the terms and conditions of the Creative Commons Attribution (CC BY) license (http://creativecommons.org/licenses/by/4.0/).

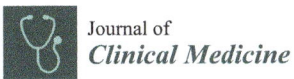

Article

Poor Efficacy of L-Acetylcarnitine in the Treatment of Asthenozoospermia in Patients with Type 1 Diabetes

Rosita A. Condorelli [1], Aldo E. Calogero [1], Rossella Cannarella [1], Filippo Giacone [1], Laura M. Mongioì [1], Laura Cimino [1], Antonio Aversa [2] and Sandro La Vignera [1,*]

1. Department of Clinical and Experimental Medicine, University of Catania, 95123 Catania, Italy; rosita.condorelli@unict.it (R.A.C.); acaloger@unict.it (A.E.C.); roxcannarella@gmail.com (R.C.); filippogiacone@yahoo.it (F.G.); lauramongioi@hotmail.it (L.M.M.); lauracimino@hotmail.it (L.C.)
2. Department of Experimental and Clinical Medicine, Magna Graecia University of Catanzaro, 88100 Catanzaro, Italy; aversa@unicz.it
* Correspondence: sandrolavignera@unict.it; Fax: ++39-095-3781180

Received: 1 April 2019; Accepted: 25 April 2019; Published: 28 April 2019

Abstract: Introduction. In recent years, research has focused on the impact that diabetes mellitus (DM) has on male reproductive function. The available evidence has mainly considered type 2 DM (DM2). However, we have previously shown that type 1 DM (DM1) also affects male reproductive health. Given the efficacy of carnitine in the treatment of male infertility, a topic that merits further investigation is its role in the treatment of infertile patients with DM1. **Aim.** To investigate the efficacy of carnitines for the treatment of asthenozoospermia in DM1 patients. **Methods.** This was a two-arm single-blind, randomized control trial. The patients enrolled in this study were assigned to the group receiving L-acetylcarnitine (LAC) (1.5 g daily for 4 months) or to the group receiving LAC (same dosage) plus L-carnitine (LC) (2 g daily for 4 months). Serum-glycated hemoglobin levels did not differ significantly after either of the two treatments given. Administration of LAC plus LC showed greater efficacy on progressive sperm motility than single therapy (increase 14% vs. 1% after treatment, respectively). **Discussion.** The results of this study showed that the administration of LAC plus LC is more effective than the administration of LAC alone. The lower efficacy of LAC alone could be due to the lower overall administered dosage. Alternatively, a selective defect of carnitine transporters at an epididymal level could be hypothesized in patients with DM1. Further studies are needed to clarify this point.

Keywords: type 1 diabetes; asthenozoospermia; carnitine

1. Introduction

In recent years, scientific interest for the potential male reproductive consequences of diabetes mellitus (DM) has been growing [1]. The greatest attention has been given to patients with type 2 DM (DM2), mainly because of its greater prevalence and clearer pathogenic mechanisms (hypogonadism, oxidative stress, neuropathy, sexual dysfunction) [1–4]. However, data concerning sperm quality also emerge in type 1 DM (DM1) patients. The latter is a disease with a different pathophysiology compared with DM2, being characterized by an absolute lack of insulin secretion compared to the condition of insulin-resistance typically found in DM2 patients [5,6]. In particular, a recent meta-analysis has shown a significant decrease in the volume of ejaculate in DM1 patients [7].

We previously reported a significant decrease in the sperm motility of DM1 patients, suggesting the need to evaluate a complication that is not usually considered. In our previous study, we showed that specific alteration of the sperm mitochondrial membrane potential in these patients occurs some years before sperm motility decline becomes evident during sperm analysis [5,6].

The pharmacological treatment of asthenozoospermia is very controversial, and hormonal and non-hormonal therapeutic options may be used. L-acetylcarnitine (LAC) and/or L-carnitine (LC) are often used in these patients. The rationale for its use is based on the potential antioxidant and prokinetic effects. Several lines of clinical evidence have been published showing different treatment protocols using single or combined strategies [8]. A recent meta-analysis of the literature has shown that LC improves sperm parameters, placing it among the treatment options for idiopathic infertility together with other possible treatments, such as pentoxifylline, coenzyme Q10, follicle-stimulating hormone, tamoxifen, and kallikrein [9].

Total and free carnitine levels have been reported to be low in patients with DM1. This decrease is related to the duration of the disease, and could potentially affect long-term complications in these patients [10–12].

The potential causes of the carnitine decrement found in DM1 patients are many. It may be due to lower dietary intake, decreased intestinal absorption, and/or increased renal excretion. At the same time, the chronic consequences associated with this deficiency are not completely known. We have no evidence regarding the consequences of this deficiency on sperm parameters or the effects of integration in DM1 patients [10–12].

Therefore, the present study was undertaken to evaluate the effects on sperm parameters of the administration of LAC alone or in combination with LC in DM1 patients with asthenozoospermia.

2. Patients and Methods

The study was conducted on 40 asthenozoospermic patients with DM1 aged 18–35 years. Patients with any of the following conditions were excluded from the study: chronic complications of diabetes (neuropathy, nephropathy, retinopathy); dyslipidemia; hypertension; body mass index ≥ 30.0 kg/m^2; presence of mono- and/or bilateral varicocele; diagnosis of male accessory gland infection/inflammation; congenital and/or acquired obstruction of proximal and/or distal seminal ducts; testicular volume <12 mL (according to Prader's orchidometer); hypogonadism, defined by total testosterone <3 ng/mL or 10.4 nM; hyperprolactinemia, defined by a level above the upper limit of normal after a single measurement of serum levels; hyperestrogenism; thyroid disorders; cryptorchidism; cigarette smoking; recent drug and/or alcohol abuse. All patients had a basal bolus scheme of insulin therapy with an exogenous insulin/body weight ratio of 0.5/kg.

Two semen samples, 2–3 weeks apart, were obtained from each patient before and after 4 months of pharmacological treatment. The mean values of both measurements were considered for the statistical analysis.

A blood sample was collected from the antecubital vein, at 08:30, to measure serum concentrations of luteinizing hormone, follicle-stimulating hormone, total testosterone, 17β-estradiol, prolactin, and glycated hemoglobin (HbA1c). HbA1C was re-evaluated after 4 months for clinical control assessment.

All patients provided written informed consent before enrollment, and were aware that their data would be used for clinical research purposes. The protocol was approved by the internal review board of Operative Unit of Andrology and Endocrinology Policlinico G. Rodolico University Hospital, Catania, Italy. (approval no. 07/2018).

Patients were divided into two groups for randomly received treatment: Group A was given LAC 500 mg tablets every 8 h every day for 4 months, and group B received the same dose of LAC plus LC 2 g oral solution once daily for 4 months. Randomization was based on a single sequence of random assignments generated from PC (simple randomization) in a single-blind procedure.

3. Sperm Analysis

Semen samples were collected by masturbation into a sterile container after 3–5 days of sexual abstinence. After liquefaction, semen was analyzed according to the World Health Organization criteria (WHO, 2010). Semen analysis was performed by the same technician (FG).

4. Measurement of Serum Hormone Concentrations

The hormone assays were performed by electrochemiluminescence with a Roche/Hitachi device (Cobas 6000; Roche Diagnostics, Indianapolis, IN, USA). The reference intervals were as follows: Luteinizing hormone 1.6–9.0 mUI mL^{-1}, Follicle Stimulating Hormone = 2.0–12.0 mUI mL^{-1}, 17β-estradiol = 8.0–43.0 pg mL^{-1}, total testosterone = 2.8–8.0 ng mL^{-1}, prolactin = 4.0–15.0 ng mL^{-1}.

5. Statistical Analysis

All statistical analyses were performed using SPSS v. 19 software (SPSS Inc, IBM Corp, Somers, NY, USA). Continuous variables, presented as median (interquartile range), were tested by Mann–Whitney U test or Kruskal–Wallis test according to their non-normal distribution (normality of variable distribution was tested by Kolmogorov–Smirnov test). A p-value lower than 0.05 was considered statistically significant. Spearman's or Pearson's correlation coefficients were used to test the associations between different variables.

6. Results

There were no drop-out patients as all completed the study protocol. Following randomization, group A and B did not differ significantly for the following parameters: age (25.0 ± 2.0 vs. 27.0 ± 2.0 years), body mass index (22.0 ± 1.0 vs. 23.0 ± 1.0 kg/m^2), disease duration (12.0 ± 2.0 vs. 14.0 ± 3.0 years), HbA1c (7.8 ± 1.2 vs. 8.1 ± 1.5 %). HbA1c values were also similar after 4 months of treatment (7.2 ± 1.3 vs. 7.4 ± 1.3 %) (Figure 1). Compared to at enrollment, HbA1c values decreased slightly in both groups, but the difference was not statistically significant. HbA1c levels did not correlate with any of the evaluated sperm parameters.

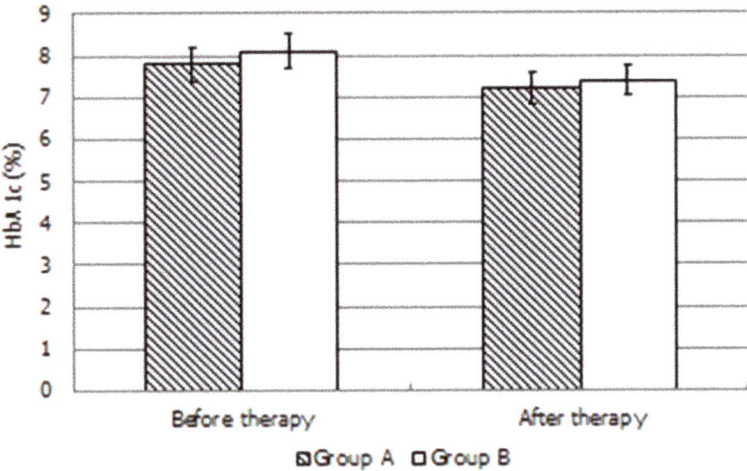

Figure 1. Glycated hemoglobin levels in each group of patients with type 1 diabetes mellitus before and after administration of L-Acetyl-Carnitine or L-Acetyl-Carnitine plus L-Carnitine. Type 1 diabetes mellitus (DM1) (a) L-acetylcarnitine (LAC) 500 mg tablets every 8 h every day for 4 months; DM (b) LAC 500 mg tablets every 8 h and LC 2 g oral solution only once a day for 4 months. Values are shown as mean ± SD.

At the time of enrollment, groups A and B did not differ in anthropometric, seminal, and hormonal parameters (Table 1). After 4 months of treatment, DM1 patients treated with LAC plus LC showed significantly higher progressive sperm motility compared with DM1 patients treated with LAC alone (Table 2 and Figure 2). In group A, after treatment, we observed a significant increase ($p < 0.05$) of progressive sperm motility in two patients (10%). In group B, 10 patients (50%) had a significant improvement ($p < 0.05$) of this parameter compared to baseline. No patient of the two groups showed a progressive motility value of >32% after therapy, a value considered to be the lower threshold for this parameter (WHO, 2010).

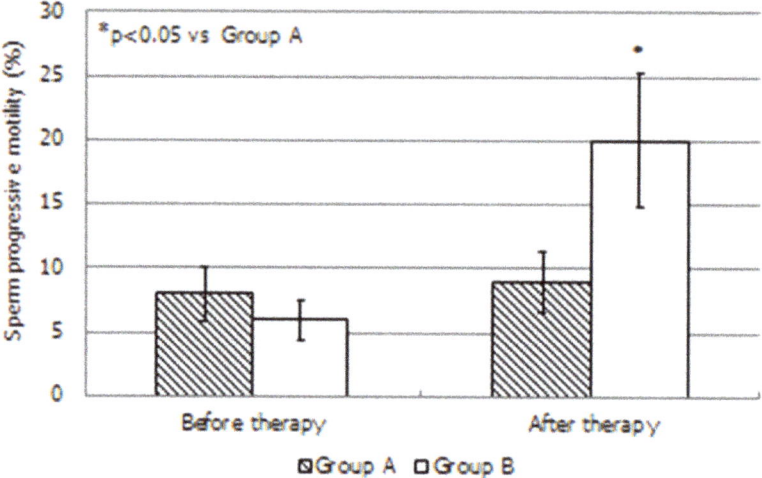

Figure 2. Sperm progressive motility in each group of patients with type 1 diabetes mellitus before and after administration of L-Acetyl-Carnitine or L-Acetyl-Carnitine plus L-Carnitine. DM1 (a) LAC 500 mg tablets every 8 h every day for 4 months; DM (b) LAC 500 mg tablets every 8 h and LC 2 g oral solution only once a day for 4 months. Values are shown as mean ± SD; * $p < 0.05$ compared to DM1 (a).

Table 1. Anthropometric, seminal, and hormonal characteristics of patients at enrollment.

Parameters	Group A (n = 20)	Group B (n = 20)	p-value
Anthropometric parameters			
Age (years), median (IQR)	25.0 (22.0–33.0)	27.0 (24.0–35.0)	0.30
Weight (kg), median (IQR)	69.0 (64.5–76.5)	71.0 (60.5–77.0)	0.69
Height (m), median (IQR)	176.0 (170.0–179.0)	174.5 (168.5–178.0)	0.30
Body mass index (kg/m^2), median (IQR)	23.0 (21.25–24.75)	24.0 (22.25–29.75)	0.30
Waist circumference (cm), median (IQR)	86.0 (81.25–88.0)	88.0 (82.0–90.0)	0.25
Sperm parameters			
Volume (mL), median (IQR)	1.8 (1.6–3.0)	1.9 (1.6–3.2)	0.97
Concentration (mil/mL), median (IQR)	25.0 (20.0–45.0)	28.0 (22.0–50.0)	0.26
Progressive motility (%), median (IQR)	8.0 (2.0–12.0)	7.0 (3.0–15.0)	0.69
Normal forms (%), median (IQR)	8.0 (6.0–14.0)	7.0 (5.0–15.0)	0.72
Leucocytes (mil/mL), median (IQR)	0.4 (0.30–0.80)	0.5 (0.2–0.8)	0.96
Hormonal parameters			
LH (UI/L), median (IQR)	2.3 (1.72–2.57)	2.1 (0.8–2.55)	0.22
FSH (UI/L), median (IQR)	2.9 (2.50–3.50)	2.6 (0.32–3.3)	0.30
TT (ng/mL), median (IQR)	6.2 (5.0–8.2)	6.4 (4.8–8.2)	0.30
E2 (pg/mL), median (IQR)	9.0 (6.25–11.5)	8.6 (5.0–13.75)	0.24
PRL (ng/mL), median (IQR)	10.5 (7.25–12.75)	12.0 (6.0–16.0)	0.26

Legend: DM1 (a) LAC 500 mg tablets every 8 h every day for 4 months; DM (b) LAC 500 mg tablets every 8 h and LC 2 gr oral solution only once a day for 4 months.

Table 2. Sperm parameters before and after 4 months of pharmacological treatment.

Parameter	Group A at Enrollment	Group A after Treatment	Group B at Enrollment	Group B after Treatment
Volume (mL), median (IQR)	1.8 (1.6–3.0)	2.0 (1.5–3.2)	1.9 (1.6–3.2)	2.3 (1.5–3.5)
Concentration (mil/mL), median (IQR)	25.0 (20.0–45.0)	29.0 (22.0–49.0)	28.0 (22.0–50.0)	32.0 (24.0–51.0)
Progressive motility (%), median (IQR)	8.0 (2.0–12.00)	9.0 (2.0–14.00)	7.0 (3.0–15.00)	20.0 * (5.0–28.00)
Normal forms (%), median (IQR)	8.0 (6.0–14.0)	10.0 (7.0–16.0)	7.0 (5.0–14.0)	11.0 (7.0–18.0)
Leucocytes (mil/mL), median (IQR)	0.4 (0.3–0.8)	0.5 (0.3–0.8)	0.5 (0.2–0.8)	0.3 (0.1–0.6)

Legend: Values of two seminal evaluations before and after pharmacological treatment. DM1 (a) LAC 500 mg tablets every 8 h every day for 4 months. DM (b) LAC 500 mg tablets every 8 h and LC 2 g oral solution only once a day for 4 months. * $p < 0.05$ compared to DM1 (a).

7. Discussion

The results of the present study showed that the administration of LAC (1.5 g daily for 4 months)—a treatment currently adopted in the andrological clinical practice to improve sperm motility [8] is not effective for the treatment of asthenozoospermia in DM1 patients. By contrast, the concomitant administration of LAC plus LC (2 g daily) to age-matched DM1 patients was shown to be efficacious in improving progressive sperm motility. After the 4-month-long administration, both groups showed a slight but no significant decrease in HbA1c levels.

Carnitine is a short-chain non-protein amino acid. It is a carrier of fatty acids, allowing mitochondria to use them for the production of Adenosin triphospfate. The fatty acids must be activated within the cytosol before being degraded. Their complete degradation then occurs in the mitochondria instead. The activated fatty acids are found in the form of acyl-CoA, a fatty acid linked to a molecule of coenzyme A. However, acyl-CoA is not able to cross the mitochondrial membrane due to the presence of its acyl portion. The acyl portion is then transferred to a carnitine molecule, forming acylcarnitine [8].

Carnitines display its positive effects on human general health, particularly in LC formulation, which is derived from endogenous synthesis and food intake. LC acts as a transporter for long-chain fatty acids into the mitochondria, in turn facilitating energy and LAC production. The latter is synthetized by the L-carnitine acetyltransferase, which is responsible for mitochondrial coenzyme A (CoA) and acyl-CoA concentrations [13–15].

The presence of a relationship between carnitine and DM has been established. Subjects of more debate are concerned with lower carnitine serum levels, their possible predictive role in the diagnosis of DM1, and efficacy in the treatment of diabetic neuropathy. In particular, several studies have highlighted decreased carnitine levels in DM1 and DM2 patients, and the reasons for this are unclear. Possible explanations may be lower absorption capacity, an unbalanced diet, or increased excretion through urine [12]. Recently, a meta-analysis carried out on four different global studies, including 284 patients, evaluated the efficacy of LC administration in DM2 patients, reporting an improvement of glycemia, total cholesterol, low-density-lipoprotein (LDL) cholesterol, B100, and A1 apolipoproteins, with a 2–3 daily administration [16]. Carnitine deficiency can hinder the entry of fatty acids into the mitochondrial membrane, leading to weight increase, low muscular tone, increased cytosolic concentration of triglycerides, excessive appetite, and glycemic fluctuations [16].

Concerning DM1, the results are promising despite the low quantities of evidence. Accordingly, carnitine deficiency in the first few days of neonatal life has been addressed as a possible cause of the development of DM1 [11]. Indeed, molecules belonging to the carnitine family remove autoreactive immune cells responsible for the disease. In summary, low carnitine levels during neonatal life may cause predisposition to DM1 [11].

Mamoulakis and colleagues (2004) highlighted the decreased total and free carnitine levels in 47 DM1 patients compared to controls, and showed a relationship with disease duration, suggesting a correlation with the complications of the disease [12].

Several lines of evidence have highlighted the neurotrophic and analgesic effects of LAC in the treatment of diabetic neuropathy. Hence, LAC is currently prescribed in the clinical practice for the treatment of this complication [17].

No data are available concerning the possible beneficial effects of carnitine in DM patients with sperm parameter abnormalities. On the contrary, a number of studies confirm carnitine pro-kinetic and antioxidant activity in male idiopathic infertility [8]. A recent meta-analysis confirms this effect while underlining two aspects: (a) limited evidence regarding pregnancy and live birth rate; (b) the controversial methodological aspects of the analyzed studies (Omar et al., 2019). Overall, the quality of the studies and the efficacy of carnitine for the treatment of idiopathic male infertility should be considered moderate.

Moncada and colleagues reported a significant improvement of sperm motility in 20 patients with idiopathic oligoasthenoteratozoospermia after the 60-day-long administration of LAC at a daily dose of 4 g [18]. In the studies by Costa et al. [19] and Vitali et al. [20] the 3 g daily administration of LC for 3–4 months was effective in ameliorating sperm motility [19,20]. Subsequently, several studies have been carried out using a combination of LC and LAC at a daily dosage of 2 and 1 g, respectively, for 3 months, or at the same dosage for six months. Finally, Balercia and colleagues (2005) adopted a therapeutic scheme of 3 g daily administration of LAC and LC for 6 months [21].

The interpretation of the results of the present study is not unique. High carnitine concentrations occur at the epididymal level. LC is actively transported into the epididymis through specific transporters known as carnitine/organic cation transporters (OCTNs). The OCTN isoform 1 (OCTN1) shows a low specificity for carnitine. On the contrary, OCTN2 has a high specificity for carnitine at the epididymal level [13–15]. No data have currently been reported on the expression of OCTNs in epididymal spermatozoa in DM, neither in animal models nor in humans. This topic deserves further investigation. It will be necessary to evaluate the existence of a selective deficit of this category to understand the differences in the efficacy of LC plus LAC compared to LAC alone on progressive sperm motility in DM1 patients.

At the same time, the LC and LAC dosage adopted in this study as well as the treatment duration may be considered insufficient when compared with previous reports of the literature [8].

Finally, further studies should be performed to investigate mitochondrial function in DM patients before starting the treatment to assess whether a low mitochondrial membrane potential may influence the effectiveness of carnitine and, in turn, the dosage to be prescribed. We have previously shown that an alteration of this parameter promotes asthenozoospermia in DM1 patients [6].

Similar considerations should also be applied to the epididymal US feature, since signs of inflammation or neuropathy on US have been revealed to promote the diagnosis [3,5].

8. Study Limitations

The main limitations of this study are the low sample size, the unavailability of biofunctional sperm parameters (mitochondrial function and α1-glycosidases levels, the latter being a marker of epididymal secretory function) as well as of the epididymal ultrasound characteristics. Another limitation concerns the lack of a true control arm (placebo) and, also, the possibility that more frequent sampling in a more extended protocol might be of interest. According to the current guidelines [22], DM1 patients are not considered at risk for infertility. Therefore, information derived from their sperm quality is important for a better understanding of biochemical mechanisms and possible future clinical applications.

Author Contributions: The conceptualization, R.A.C. and S.L.V.; methodology, R.A.C., S.L.V., F.G.; software, R.C.; validation, A.E.C., A.A.; formal analysis, S.L.V., A.E.C.; investigation, L.C., L.M.M., F.G., R.C.; writing—review and editing, S.L.V., R.A.C., A.A., A.E.C.

Conflicts of Interest: The authors declare no conflict of interest.

References

1. La Vignera, S.; Condorelli, R.; Vicari, E.; D'Agata, R. Calogero AE. Diabetes mellitus and sperm parameters. *J. Androl.* **2012**, *33*, 145–153. [CrossRef]
2. Condorelli, R.A.; Calogero, A.E.; Vicari, E.; Duca, Y.; Favilla, V.; Morgia, G.; Cimino, S.; Di Mauro, M.; La Vignera, S. Prevalence of male accessory gland inflammations/infections in patients with Type 2 diabetes mellitus. *J. Endocrinol. Invest.* **2013**, *36*, 770–774.
3. Condorelli, R.A.; Vicari, E.; Calogero, A.E.; La Vignera, S. Male accessory gland inflammation prevalence in type 2 diabetic patients with symptoms possibly reflecting autonomic neuropathy. *Asian J. Androl.* **2014**, *16*, 761–766. [PubMed]
4. La Vignera, S.; Condorelli, R.A.; Vicari, E.; D'Agata, R.; Salemi, M.; Calogero, A.E. High levels of lipid peroxidation in semen of diabetic patients. *Andrologia* **2012**, *44*, 565–570. [CrossRef] [PubMed]
5. Condorelli, R.A.; La Vignera, S.; Mongioì, L.M.; Alamo, A.; Calogero, A.E. Diabetes Mellitus and Infertility: Different Pathophysiological Effects in Type 1 and Type 2 on Sperm Function. *Front. Endocrinol. (Lausanne).* **2018**, *9*, 268. [CrossRef]
6. La Vignera, S.; Condorelli, R.A.; Di Mauro, M.; Lo Presti, D.; Mongioì, L.M.; Russo, G.; Calogero, A.E. Reproductive function in male patients with type 1 diabetes mellitus. *Andrology* **2015**, *3*, 1082–1087. [CrossRef] [PubMed]
7. Pergialiotis, V.; Prodromidou, A.; Frountzas, M.; Korou, L.M.; Vlachos, G.D.; Perrea, D. Diabetes mellitus and functional sperm characteristics: A meta-analysis of observational studies. *J. Diabetes Complications.* **2016**, *30*, 1167–1176. [CrossRef] [PubMed]
8. Mongioi', L.; Calogero, A.E.; Vicari, E.; Condorelli, R.A.; Russo, G.I.; Privitera, S.; Morgia, G.; La Vignera, S. The role of carnitine in male infertility. *Andrology* **2016**, *4*, 800–807. [CrossRef]
9. Omar, M.I.; Pal, R.P.; Kelly, B.D.; Bruins, H.M.; Yuan, Y.; Diemer, T.; Krausz, C.; Tournaye, H.; Kopa, Z.; Jungwirth, A.; et al. Benefits of Empiric Nutritional and Medical Therapy for Semen Parameters and Pregnancy and Live Birth Rates in Couples with Idiopathic Infertility: A Systematic Review and Meta-analysis. *Eur. Urol.* **2019**, *75*, 615–625. [CrossRef] [PubMed]
10. Coker, M.; Coker, C.; Darcan, S.; Can, S.; Orbak, Z.; Gökşen, D. Carnitine metabolism in diabetes mellitus. *J. Pediatr. Endocrinol. Metab.* **2002**, *15*, 841–849. [CrossRef] [PubMed]
11. La Marca, G.; Malvagia, S.; Toni, S.; Piccini, B.; Di Ciommo, V.; Bottazzo, G.F. Children who develop type 1 diabetes early in life show low levels of carnitine and amino acids at birth: Does this finding shed light on the etiopathogenesis of the disease? *Nutr. Diabetes.* **2013**, *28*, e94. [CrossRef] [PubMed]
12. Mamoulakis, D.; Galanakis, E.; Dionyssopoulou, E.; Evangeliou, A.; Sbyrakis, S. Carnitine deficiency in children and adolescents with type 1 diabetes. *J. Diabetes Complications.* **2004**, *18*, 271–274. [CrossRef]
13. Agarwal, A.; Said, T.M. Carnitines and male infertility. *Reprod. Biomed. Online* **2004**, *8*, 376–384. [CrossRef]
14. Lenzi, A.; Lombardo, F.; Gandini, L.; Dondero, F. Metabolism and action of L-carnitine: Its possible role in sperm tail function. *Arch. Ital. Urol. Nefrol. Androl.* **1992**, *64*, 187–196.
15. Ng, C.M.; Blackman, M.R.; Wang, C.; Swerdloff, R.S. The role of carnitine in the male reproductive system. *Ann. N.Y. Acad. Sci.* **2004**, *1033*, 177–188. [CrossRef] [PubMed]
16. Vidal-Casariego, A.; Burgos-Peláez, R.; Martínez-Faedo, C.; Calvo-Gracia, F.; Valero-Zanuy, M.Á.; Luengo-Pérez, L.M.; Cuerda-Compés, C. Metabolic effects of L-carnitine on type 2 diabetes mellitus: Systematic review and meta-analysis. *Exp. Clin. Endocrinol. Diabetes.* **2013**, *121*, 234–238. [CrossRef] [PubMed]
17. Evans, J.D.; Jacobs, T.F.; Evans, E.W. Role of acetyl-L-carnitine in the treatment of diabetic peripheral neuropathy. *Ann. Pharmacother.* **2008**, *42*, 1686–1691. [CrossRef]
18. Moncada, M.L.; Vicari, E.; Cimino, C.; Calogero, A.E.; Mongioì, A.; D'Agata, R. Effect of acetylcarnitine treatment in oligoasthenospermic patients. *Acta. Eur. Fertil.* **1992**, *23*, 221–224.

19. Costa, M.; Canale, D.; Filicori, M.; D'Iddio, S.; Lenzi, A. L-carnitine in idiopathic asthenozoospermia: A multicenter study. Italian Study Group on Carnitine and Male Infertility. *Andrologia* **1994**, *26*, 155–159. [CrossRef] [PubMed]
20. Vitali, G.; Parente, R.; Melotti, C. Carnitine supplementation in human idiopathic asthenospermia: Clinical results. *Drugs Exp. Clin. Res.* **1995**, *21*, 157–159.
21. Balercia, G.; Regoli, F.; Armeni, T.; Koverech, A.; Mantero, F.; Boscaro, M. Placebo-controlled double-blind randomized trial on the use of L-carnitine, L-acetylcarnitine, or combined L-carnitine and L-acetylcarnitine in men with idiopathic asthenozoospermia. *Fertil. Steril.* **2005**, *84*, 662–671. [CrossRef] [PubMed]
22. Ring, J.D.; Lwin, A.A.; Köhler, T.S. Current medical management of endocrine-related male infertility. *Asian J. Androl.* **2016**, *18*, 357–363. [CrossRef] [PubMed]

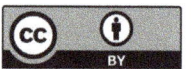

© 2019 by the authors. Licensee MDPI, Basel, Switzerland. This article is an open access article distributed under the terms and conditions of the Creative Commons Attribution (CC BY) license (http://creativecommons.org/licenses/by/4.0/).

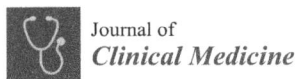

Review

Management and Treatment of Varicocele in Children and Adolescents: An Endocrinologic Perspective

Rossella Cannarella [1], Aldo E. Calogero [1], Rosita A. Condorelli [1], Filippo Giacone [1], Antonio Aversa [2] and Sandro La Vignera [1,*]

[1] Department of Clinical and Experimental Medicine, University of Catania, 95125 Catania, Italy
[2] Department of Experimental and Clinical Medicine, University Magna Graecia of Catanzaro, 88100 Catanzaro, Italy
* Correspondence: sandrolavignera@unict.it; Tel.: +39-95-3782311

Received: 8 July 2019; Accepted: 3 September 2019; Published: 8 September 2019

Abstract: Pediatric varicocele has an overall prevalence of 15%, being more frequent as puberty begins. It can damage testicular function, interfering with Sertoli cell proliferation and hormone secretion, testicular growth and spermatogenesis. Proper management has a pivotal role for future fertility preservation. The aim of this review was to discuss the diagnosis, management and treatment of childhood and adolescent varicocele from an endocrinologic perspective, illustrating the current evidence of the European Society of Pediatric Urology (ESPU), the European Association of Urology (EAU), the American Urological Association (AUA) and the American Society for Reproductive Medicine (ASRM) scientific societies. According to the ASRM/ESPU/AUA practice committee, the treatment of adolescent varicocele is indicated in the case of decreased testicular volume or sperm abnormalities, while it is contraindicated in subclinical varicocele. The recent EAS/ESPU meta-analysis reports that moderate evidence exists on the benefits of varicocele treatment in children and adolescents in terms of testicular volume and sperm concentration increase. No specific phenotype in terms of testicular volume cut-off or peak retrograde flow (PRF) is indicated. Based on current evidence, we suggest that conservative management may be suggested in patients with PRF < 30 cm/s, testicular asymmetry < 10% and no evidence of sperm and hormonal abnormalities. In patients with 10–20% testicular volume asymmetry or 30 < PRF ≤ 38 cm/s or sperm abnormalities, careful follow-up may ensue. In the case of absent catch-up growth or sperm recovery, varicocele repair should be suggested. Finally, treatment can be proposed at the initial consultation in painful varicocele, testicular volume asymmetry ≥ 20%, PRF > 38 cm/s, infertility and failure of testicular development.

Keywords: pediatric varicocele; testicular volume asymmetry; peak retrograde flow; varicocele repair

1. Introduction

Testicular varicocele is defined by the abnormal dilation and tortuosity of the pampiniform plexus draining the testes. The prevalence of varicocele is a debated issue since it depends on the selected population (infertile, fertile, age of patients) or the methods used to make the diagnosis (clinical examination and/or Doppler ultrasound). Most of the early epidemiological studies reported that the prevalence of varicocele in the general male adult population is approximately 15%, despite more recent studies suggesting the occurrence of an age-related prevalence or that it is inversely correlated with the body mass index. The prevalence of varicocele also seems to differ among fertile and infertile men or in those with primary or secondary infertility [1].

The prevalence in childhood and adolescence mirrors that in adulthood. Recently, a European study carried out in 7000 young men (median age: 19 years) reported the occurrence of varicocele in 15.7% of cases [2]. In a cohort of 4052 Turkish children and adolescents, its prevalence was 0.8% in

2–6-year-old boys, 1% in 7–10-year-old boys, 7.8 in 11–14-year-old boys, and 14.1% in 15–19-year-old boys [3], indicating an increasing prevalence as puberty begins.

Several data, mainly obtained from the adult population, suggest that varicocele has a negative role on testicular function. Accordingly, poorer semen quality and pregnancy outcomes have been reported in patients with varicocele compared to healthy controls [4–6]. In agreement, varicocele repair has been shown to improve both conventional (sperm concentration, progressive motility and normal forms) and bio-functional sperm parameters (percentage of spermatozoa with low mitochondrial membrane potential, phosphatidylserine externalization, abnormal chromatin compactness and DNA fragmentation) [4,6] and the outcome of assisted reproductive techniques (ARTs) [5]. In particular, the best quality of evidence comes from a meta-analysis provided by the American Society for Reproductive Medicine (ASRM) performed on 1241 patients with oligozoospermia or azoospermia and a history of varicocele undergoing ART. Pregnancy, live birth and sperm extraction rates were assessed following varicocele repair. Treatment led to improvement in pregnancy and live birth rates in oligozoospermic (odds ratio (OR) 1.699 and 2.366) and combined oligospermic/azoospermic patients (OR 1.761 and 1.760) compared to untreated patients. In addition, the live birth rate was higher in patients undergoing intra-uterine insemination (IUI) (OR 8.36). Similarly, the sperm retrieval rate increased after varicocele repair in azoospermic patients (OR 2.509). Based on such evidence, varicocele repair should be considered as a treatment option in oligozoospermic or azoospermic patients before they undergo ART [5]. Interestingly, the negative impact of varicocele on testicular function might also be extended to the Leydig cells. Indeed, according to meta-analytic data, its repair resulted in an increase in testosterone levels by 97.48 ng/dL [7].

The consequences of varicocele on testicular function in childhood and adolescence have been investigated to a lesser extent. In the last decade, a consensus was reached on the conditions requiring varicocele repair in adulthood [8]. On the contrary, several aspects of the management and treatment of varicocele in childhood and adolescence are poorly defined and still debated.

Adolescents with varicocele are highly heterogeneous, due to rapid changes in hormone levels and the stage of pubertal development [9]. This makes a standard approach more difficult. The current challenge is to establish which patient should be treated, when and what type of treatment should be preferred [10].

The aim of this review was to discuss the impact of varicocele on testicular function in childhood and adolescence from an endocrinological perspective and to highlight the best practice in diagnosis, management and treatment, according to the established guidelines by the European Society of Pediatric Urology (ESPU), European Association of Urology (EAU), the American Urological Association (AUA) and the ASRM.

To accomplish this, an extensive search in PubMed, Embase and Cochrane Library was performed by two independent authors (RC and RAC) using the following key-words: "varicocele", "childhood", "adolescent", "diagnosis", "management", "treatment", "sperm analysis", "testicular volume", "AMH", "Inhibin B", "nutcracker". Only English language studies published from each database inception up to 30 July 2019 have been included. In addition, reference lists form articles were searched. No restriction on study design was used.

2. Pathogenesis of Testicular Damage

The evidence collected in children and adolescents suggests a negative impact of varicocele on testicular function, including sperm abnormalities, testicular hypotrophy and hormone alterations.

In more detail, varicocele is able to alter the conventional semen parameters in youth. A meta-analysis carried out in 357 patients with varicocele aged 15–24 years reported a statistically significant decrease in sperm concentration (−24 million/mL), motility (−7.5%) and morphology (−1.7%) compared to 427 age-matched controls [11]. Reflecting the findings in adulthood [4–6], its repair led to a significant improvement in sperm concentration and motility by 14.6×10^6/mL (95% CI

(7.1–22.1 10^6/mL)) and 6.6% (95% CI (2.1–11.2%)), respectively, as shown by the same meta-analysis, suggesting a role of varicocele in the pathogenesis of sperm abnormalities [11].

Other data support these findings and indicate a role for varicocele-induced testicular hypotrophy in the establishment of sperm abnormalities. A study carried out in 57 Tanner stage V adolescent males at 14 to 20 years found that patients with testicular volume asymmetry greater than 10% had lower sperm concentrations and total motile sperm counts compared to those with asymmetry lower than 10%. A greater decrease was found in patients with a differential greater than 20% [12]. Precisely, total motile sperm counts of 64, 32 and 10 million in patients with 10%, 15% and 20% testicular asymmetry have been reported [12].

Large epidemiologic data on 7035 young men with a median age of 19 years showed that the sperm concentration halved in patients with grade III varicocele compared with healthy controls. Interestingly, patients with varicocele had higher serum levels of follicle-stimulating hormone (FSH), lower inhibin B and higher levels of luteinizing hormone (LH) compared to controls [2]. Accordingly, a study carried out in 31 pre-pubertal patients with left and nine with bilateral varicocele with an average age of 12.55 years found an increase in inhibin B levels 12 and 26 weeks after varicocele repair and a negative correlation between inhibin B and FSH serum levels [13]. Taken together, these findings suggest the occurrence of a Sertoli cell dysfunction in adolescent patients with varicocele, since inhibin B is secreted by these cells. This information is of particular interest for the assessment of testicular function in young patients, when sperm parameters cannot be evaluated.

The exact mechanisms by which varicocele can damage testicular function are not entirely clear. Several theories have been suggested so far.

Varicocele causes scrotal hyperthermia, which has a deleterious effect on spermatogenesis. Genetic factors play a role in the pathogenesis of varicocele, as it has a higher prevalence in first-degree relatives of men with known varicocele compared to controls [14] and also seems to be involved in the predisposition of varicocele-induced testicular damage. Accordingly, the genetically decreased expression of the heat-shock-proteins (HSPs) can contribute to heat stress, which, in turn, is associated with the markers of oxidative stress (OS) and apoptosis [15]. Transient exposure to high temperatures can reduce testis weight by interfering with spermatogenesis. In addition, blood stasis in varicose veins promotes leucocyte trapping, reactive oxygen species (ROS) overproduction and can cause testicular hypoxia. Low anti-apoptotic and increased pro-apoptotic gene expression (*HSP*, *Metallothireonin-1*, *BCL-2*, *BAX*, *PHUDA1*, *PRM2*, and *CCIN*) may confer susceptibility to OS and thermogenic damage, thus explaining the reason why high-degree varicocele does not always cause testicular damage [15].

Testes mainly consist of immature Sertoli cells which undergo proliferation and secrete the anti-Müllerian hormone (AMH) in childhood. In this phase, testicular volume reflects Sertoli cell proliferation. When puberty starts, Sertoli cells move from an immature to a mature state and lose the ability to proliferate. The final number of Sertoli cells reached at puberty will condition the spermatogenetic potential, since each Sertoli cell can support a defined number of germ cells [16].

Any event able to interfere with Sertoli cell proliferation in childhood may potentially impair testicular volume and the spermatogenetic potential in adolescence and adulthood. Importantly, a high temperature is able to affect Sertoli cell proliferation [17]. As a consequence, varicocele may hypothetically impact on the final Sertoli cell number in childhood (at least in some cases), thus inducing damage that cannot be reverted later in life. This highlights the importance of proper management and treatment in childhood/adolescence.

3. Evaluation

Adolescent varicocele is more frequently asymptomatic, despite chronic fullness or swelling in the scrotum or the inguinal area can be reported by the patient [10]. It is more frequently left sided, mainly due to the anatomical differences between left and right venous drainage. Testicular venous drainage enters the left renal vein at a sharp 90° angle. By contrast, it directly enters into the inferior vena cava in the right side. Also, the route of the left spermatic vein is longer than that of the right side.

Furthermore, the left renal vein is compressed through the angle between the abdominal aorta and the superior mesenteric artery, when flowing into the inferior vena cava. These factors cause increased pressure in the left scrotum vein, leading to varicose veins occurrence [18]. A total of 3% are bilaterally palpable [10,19].

In most cases, adolescent varicocele is diagnosed during routine medical examination for school or sports or by testicular self-examination. Physical examination is the first step for the diagnosis of varicocele. It must be performed in the supine position for scrotum and genital inspection and for the palpation of testes, epididymis and deferent ducts. Testicular consistence must be appreciated, and the volume should be evaluated by Prader's orchidometer, taking into consideration that it can overestimate the real value. The patient has to be asked to perform a Valsalva's maneuver in the standing position. Varicocele usually presents as a plexus of veins with the consistency of a "bag of worms". Clinical stadiation can be performed using the Dubin and Amelar system: grade 0 identifies subclinical varicocele (not clinically detectable, hence identified by ultrasound); grade I, which is palpable only during the Valsalva maneuver; grade II, appreciable also without the Valsalva maneuver; grade III, detected at inspection [20].

Scrotal ultrasound precisely evaluates testicular volume, the value of which is important when deciding whether varicocele repair is needed. It can be computed using the ellipsoid formula (length × width × thickness × 0.52), as described elsewhere [21]. Doppler ultrasound efficaciously indicates the varicocele grade, providing information on the maximum vein diameter and on the peak retrograde flow (PRF). In particular, varicocele is defined by the presence of multiple veins greater than 3.0–3.5 mm with concomitant retrograde blood flow. Reflux is classified as grade I (brief) when it lasts less than 1 s; grade II (intermediate) for 1–2 s and decreasing during the Valsalva maneuver and completely disappearing before the end of the maneuver; grade III (permanent) for reflux lasting more than 2 s and exhibiting a plateau aspect during the Valsalva maneuver [6]. Several scales are currently available to estimate the severity of varicocele. The most adopted ones are those developed by Sarteschi and by Dubin. The first, made of five different degrees, requires the patient to be lying down and standing. The Dubin scale includes three stages and is performed in the supine position [22]. These classifications are summarized in Table 1.

Table 1. Ultrasound varicocele degree classifications.

Scale	Degree	Description
Sarteschi	I	Reflux detected only during the Valsalva maneuver, in the absence of evident scrotal varicosity during US study.
	II	Small posterior varicosity that extends to the superior pole of the testes. Their diameter increases and the reflux becomes detectable in the supratesticular region only during the Valsalva maneuver.
	III	Vessels appear enlarged in the superior pole only in the standing position. No enlargement can be detected in the supine position. Reflux is observed only during the Valsalva maneuver.
	IV	Vessels appear enlarged in the supine position. Dilatation is more marked during the Valsalva maneuver.
	V	Venus ectasia is detected in the prone and supine position. Reflux occurs at rest and it does not increase during the Valsalva maneuver.
Dubin	0	Moderate and transient venous reflux during the Valsalva maneuver.
	I	Persistent venous reflux that ends before the Valsalva maneuver is completed.
	II	Persistent venous reflux through the entire Valsalva maneuver.
	III	Venous reflux is basally detected and does not change during the Valsalva manuever

Patients exhibiting abnormally high venous velocity ratios should be evaluated for the nutcracker phenomenon (NcP) by Doppler ultrasound of renal vessels. The NcP is defined by compression of the left renal vein between the aorta and the mesentery artery. This causes renal venous hypertension and the dilatation of collateral veins, thus predisposing to varicocele. Recently, ultrasound criteria suggestive for the NcP have been proposed. These include a reduced aortic/superior mesenteric artery angle (normal values: 38–65 degrees), left renal vein compression at the origin of the aorta and superior mesenteric artery, increased flow velocity at the left renal vein, and left-sided varicocele with a vein lumen diameter > 3 mm [23]. Few studies have been developed on the NcP in youth. According to recent data, the NcP seems common among adolescents. In a cohort of 182 adolescents with clinical varicocele, the NcP was diagnosed in 77 patients (56.2%) who experienced higher velocity ratios than those without. In this cohort, the NcP has not been found to influence testicular asymmetry and initial or re-operative surgery [24].

Elastosonography is a non-invasive technique assessing testicular elasticity. It has already been used in undescended pediatric testes or adult varicocele. The prognostic value of elastosonography in adolescent varicocele has been recently investigated. Among a cohort of 30 patients with a clinically left varicocele, a significant change in testicular elasticity was found only in the case of volume asymmetry > 20% [25]. Currently, this technique is not routinely used in adolescents with varicocele.

Sperm analysis is an exam of pivotal importance. It has to be requested taking into account that the first ejaculation usually occurs 1.5 years after the onset of puberty [26]. Worryingly, it is not widely requested by pediatrics. A 2016 survey reported that only 13% of American pediatric urologists routinely evaluated sperm analysis in adolescent patients with varicocele. A total of 50% of them had some degree of discomfort in requesting this exam and discussing semen collection with patients so young [27]. This is alarming considering that several data confirm the negative impact of varicocele on sperm parameters in adolescence. Accordingly, a decreased total sperm count was found in 17–20-year-old patients with left varicocele and testicular ipsilateral hypotrophy [28]. Reduced sperm motility, vitality and morphology has also been reported in patients of 17–19 years with varicocele compared to age-matched controls [29]. Furthermore, sperm motility was profoundly more affected as basal blood flow velocity, maximal blood flow velocity, and pampiniform vein diameter increase [29]. In addition, a study carried out on 57 Tanner V patients (14–20 years old) reported lower sperm concentrations and total motile sperm counts in patients with a testicular differential > 10% compared to those with a differential < 10%. This was even more evident where the asymmetry > 20%, showing this group had a total motile sperm count < 10 million [12].

Despite the lack of consensus, the hormone profile may be useful for the workup of adolescent varicocele, since higher levels of FSH and LH and lower levels of inhibin B have been reported [2]. Other evidence confirmed the decrease in inhibin B levels, but not gonadotropin alteration [30]. AMH and inhibin B may be of particular utility when puberty is not already started and sperm analysis cannot be performed, especially when gonadotropin and testosterone levels are still not indicative. The testes have been considered silent in childhood for long. However, they secrete AMH and inhibin B in this phase. Particularly, serum AMH and inhibin B levels have already been suggested as markers of testicular function in pre-pubertal age [15]. Accordingly, impaired AMH and inhibin B levels have been reported in prepubertal and pubertal boys with varicocele [13,31].

4. Management

The management of childhood and adolescent varicocele is still controversial since no clear consensus has been reached so far. Spontaneous catch-up growth and sperm recovery has been observed in patients with varicocele, thus suggesting that its repair is not always necessary, but conservative management consisting of monitoring and follow-up can be suggested in selected cases. The challenge is to identify accurate predictive markers which can help to select those patients who will benefit from varicocele repair.

Conservative management has been suggested in Tanner V patients with no painful varicocele and normal testicular volume. A retrospective analysis of data from 216 patients with these clinical features showed a decreased total motile sperm count (< 20 million) in 45% of cases, with a spontaneous recovery in approximately 50% of patients with poor sperm parameters at baseline [32]. Overall, this indicates a lack of sperm recovery in 22.5% of cases with no painful varicocele and normal testicular volume. No additional marker was used in this study to characterize these patients [32].

Testicular asymmetry is one parameter that has been included in the decisional flowchart. Patients with values higher than 15%–20% have historically been treated with surgery. However, in 85% of adolescents with a > 15% testicular asymmetry catch-up, growth occurs without any intervention [33]. Hence, 2–3 testicular volume measurements at different follow-up times should be reasonably performed prior to deciding on varicocele repair [33], which may be suggested in the case of failure of testicular catch-up growth.

Another important parameter is the PRF, which has been suggested as a predictor of persistent or worsening testicular asymmetry in adolescent varicocele. After a 13.2 month-long follow-up, a study carried out in a cohort of 77 patients (age range: 9 to 20 years) revealed progressive asymmetry on follow-up examination in those with ≥ 20% asymmetry or PRF ≥ 38 cm/s. On this basis, patients presenting with these parameters should undergo varicocele repair after the initial consultation. On the contrary, those with PRF < 30 cm/s are less likely to require surgery and should be carefully monitored [34]. To raise the accuracy of predictive prognostic markers, a pilot study combining testicular volume asymmetry with PRF values showed that future worsening asymmetry was associated with ≥ 20% asymmetry and PRF > 38 cm/s (the so called "20/38 harbinger"). Accordingly, 94% of patients with the 20/38 harbinger did not have catch-up growth after a 15.5 month surveillance. Hence, intervention and not surveillance should be required in this set of patients [35,36]. In patients with borderline asymmetry or PRF, intervention has been suggested in the case of the abnormality of sperm parameters [37].

To summarize, "at-risk" patients deserving consideration for intervention are those presenting the following signs and symptoms [19]: (a) persistent abnormal sperm parameters with no evidence of recovery after surveillance; (b) pain; (c) persistently altered testicular volume asymmetry with a difference > 15–20% with no evidence of catch-up growth after surveillance; (d) PRF > 38 cm/s; (e) failure of testicular development; (f) 20/38 harbinger (which can also be considered to 15/38). Decreased AMH levels in children with varicocele may need careful surveillance due to the likely occurrence of Sertoli cell dysfunction. Prospective studies are needed to confirm this.

5. Treatment Options

Several treatment options are available for varicocele repair, including surgical (e.g., open inguinal-Ivanissevich, high retroperitoneal-Palomo, subinguinal, high inguinal, microsurgical-inguinal and subinguinal, laparoscopic) and radiological (sclerotherapy, embolization, antegrade vs. retrograde) approaches.

Overall, four meta-analyses have evaluated the effects of varicocele repair in childhood and adolescence so far [11,38–40]. Zhou and collaborators [38] reported an improvement in the bilateral testicular volume following varicocelectomy compared with observation, although no benefit on sperm parameters was found. By contrast, Nork and colleagues [11] observed a moderate improvement in sperm parameters. In greater detail, data collected from 357 patients with varicocele and 427 controls showed the presence of a significantly lower sperm concentration, motility and morphology. Studies where varicocele repair was performed by "Palomo" (open or laparoscopic) technique ($n = 5$), scleroembolization ($n = 1$), inguinal or sub-inguinal intervention with magnification ($n = 4$) were included to evaluate the effect of the treatment. Varicocele repair improved sperm concentration and motility. Each technique was effective in ameliorating the sperm outcome, despite scleroembolization only being used in a single study [11].

However, the above-mentioned meta-analyses [11,38] were biased by the inclusion of non-randomized comparative studies (NCTs), thus affecting the level of evidence. Locke and colleagues [39] compared testicular volume and sperm parameters in children and adolescents (up to 21 years old) with varicocele receiving surgical or radiological intervention with those receiving no treatment. By the inclusion of only randomized comparative studies (RCTs), they showed an improvement in testicular volume (mean difference 3.18 mL) and sperm count (mean difference 25.54×10^6/mL) in treated patients compared with those undergoing conservative management. Overall, these data suggest the benefit of varicocele repair in childhood and adolescence. Nevertheless, this study [39] did not provide any information concerning a comparison of treatment options, surgical success, hydrocele formation, complication rates and paternity in the long term.

The best quality of evidence is offered by the latest systematic review and meta-analysis provided by the EAS/ESPU societies [40], including 12 RCTs (which were meta-analyzed), 47 NCTs (seven prospective and 40 retrospective) and 39 case series (which were qualitatively reviewed), for a total of 16,130 children and adolescents ≤ 21 years of age. The outcomes assessed were a short-term cure or success (evaluated < 9 months), testicular catch-up growth, pain resolution, sperm parameters and paternity (evaluated > 12 months) for benefits, complications such as testicular atrophy, hydrocele, wound infection, and failure rate for harms.

The success rate (disappearance of varicocele) was between 87% and 100% among RCTs. No difference was found neither between open and laparoscopic technique [41] nor between subinguinal and high inguinal varicocelectomy [42]. Similarly, the success rates were between 88.2% and 100% in the included NCTs and between 85.1% and 100% in the case series. Due to the lack of comparative data, no conclusion could be made concerning the type of treatment among these kinds of studies [40].

The available RCTs have assessed testicular catch-up growth in treated vs. untreated patients [43–46]. The majority of them compared inguinal and high inguinal varicocelectomy vs. observation. Only one RCT evaluated scleroembolization vs. observation [43]. Testicular volumes were significantly higher in the treated vs. untreated group (OR 1.52). NCTs report a testicular catch-up growth rate between 86 and 100% following embolization and between 62.8% and 97.1% following open varicocelectomy [40].

Data on sperm parameters coming from two RCTs [43,46] showed a significantly higher sperm concentration (mean difference 25.54×10^6/mL) in treated vs. untreated groups, in the absence of any difference in sperm motility and morphology [40]. Overall, NCTs report an improvement in sperm parameters following surgical treatment, with a follow-up ranging between 17.6 months and 10.6 years. Similar data were reported in case series [40].

Although paternity rate is one of the most important outcomes, it is rarely reported due to the necessity of long-term follow-up. The study by Cayan and colleagues [47] assessed 286 patients and 122 controls. Patients were treated by microsurgical varicocelectomy. The paternity rate was 77.3% vs. 48.4% (treated vs. untreated) leading the authors to conclude the benefit of treatment in adolescent varicocele. By contrast, the study by Bogaert et al. [48], carried out in 661 boys (12 to 17 years old) with varicocele, showed no efficacy of sclerotherapy on change in paternity as adults. Accordingly, among the 361 respondents, 158 (43%) searched for paternity, which was achieved in 85% of the conservatively followed group and 78% of the active treatment group ($p > 0.05$).

The available evidence on the onset of harms coming from RCTs suggests a resolution of pain or recurrence of pain after treatment (laparoscopic varicocelectomy), despite only two RCTs mentioning this outcome [41,42], being diminished in up to 100% of patients [42]. Post-operative (both surgical and radiological) pain resolution rates reported in NCTs were 92.9% and 100% [40]. The most common complication reported was hydrocele, and atrophy, wound infection, hematomas, scrotal emphysema and shoulder pain were observed to a lesser extent. The rate of hydrocele formation 6–85 months post-varicocelectomy was 0–12%, being the lymphatic sparing surgery associated with a lower risk compared to the non-sparing one (OR 0.08) [40].

Generally, there is moderate evidence on the benefits of varicocele repair in children and adolescents, especially in those with high-grade varicocele, low left testicular volume, pain and poor sperm parameters. However, the superiority of a specific treatment approach cannot be identified [40]. Notably, while a radiological approach represents a valid technique, the long-term risk of radiation exposure in pediatric and adolescent population following percutaneous embolization procedure should be considered.

Finally, alternative strategies (e.g., anastomosis of the proximal part of the spermatic vein with the inferior epigastric vein) could be considered in the NcP [49].

6. Established Guidelines and Societies' Positions

No guideline specifically deals with the management and treatment of childhood and adolescent varicocele. Current knowledge is extrapolated from guidelines endorsing the management of male infertility. Specifically, the ASRM/SMRU/AUA practice committee [50] suggests that varicocele diagnosis is made by th Dubin and Amelar clinical classification and to perform Doppler ultrasound only in case it is inconclusive. The treatment of adolescent varicocele is indicated in the case of decreased testicular volume or sperm abnormalities, while it is contraindicated in subclinical varicocele. The cut-off of testicular volume to suggest varicocele repair is not indicated and no specific treatment is recommended. Finally, these guidelines indicate to follow-up at least annually.

The EAU guidelines on male infertility [51] accordingly suggest using the Dubin and Amelar clinical grading classification and scrotal ultrasound to confirm the clinical findings. Worryingly, despite the authors stating that adolescent varicocele is often overtreated, no specific indication for the management and treatment of adolescent varicocele is provided. In contrast to the EAU guidelines, the EAS/ESPU meta-analysis [40] reported moderate evidence on the benefits of varicocele treatment in children and adolescents in terms of testicular volume and sperm concentration recovery. Accordingly, an ASRM society meta-analysis supports the efficacy of varicocele repair in youth on sperm concentration and motility [11].

7. Conclusions and Authors' Recommendations

Varicocele evaluation has to be clinically performed using the Dubin and Amelar scale at first. Scrotal ultrasound should be requested to precisely define testicular asymmetry and PRF. Hormone detection (including AMH and inhibin B in childhood and LH, FSH and total testosterone in adolescence) should be carried out for a comprehensive evaluation of testicular function. Importantly, sperm analysis is of pivotal importance and it may be requested at least 1.5 years after the onset of puberty. Doppler ultrasound of renal vessels should be performed in selected cases (e.g., left-sided varicocele with a vein lumen diameter > 3 mm, hematuria, proteinuria, left-sided flank/lower abdominal pain, varicose veins, urinary frequency) [23].

Current evidence clearly indicates the impact of childhood and adolescent varicocele in testicular growth and sperm output. Spontaneous testicular catch-up growth can be observed in some cases. Some markers may be used to select patients who will benefit from varicocele repair. These mainly include testicular volume asymmetry and PRF. Therefore, we suggest that conservative management could be pursued in patients with PRF < 30 cm/s, testicular asymmetry < 10% and no evidence of sperm and hormonal abnormalities. In patients with 10–20% testicular volume asymmetry or 30 < PRF ≤ 38 cm/s or sperm abnormalities, careful follow-up is advisable. In the case of absent catch-up growth or sperm recovery, varicocele repair should be suggested. Finally, treatment can be proposed at the initial consultation in painful varicocele, testicular volume asymmetry ≥ 20%, PRF > 38 cm/s, infertility and failure of testicular development. On the basis of the current evidence, either radiological or surgical intervention may be prescribed (Figure 1).

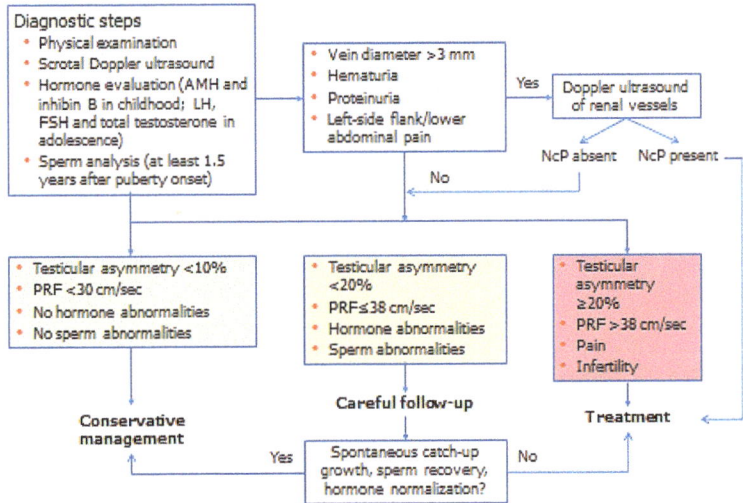

Figure 1. Management of childhood and adolescent varicocele.

Author Contributions: Conceptualization, S.L.V. and R.C.; methodology, R.A.C.; investigation, F.G.; writing—original draft preparation, R.C.; writing—review and editing, A.E.C.; visualization, S.L.V.; supervision, A.A.; project administration, A.E.C. and S.L.V.

Conflicts of Interest: The authors declare no conflict of interest.

References

1. Alsaikhan, B.; Alrabeeah, K.; Delouya, G.; Zini, A. Epidemiology of varicocele. *Asian J. Androl.* **2016**, *18*, 179–181. [PubMed]
2. Damsgaard, J.; Joensen, U.N.; Carlsen, E.; Erenpreiss, J.; Blomberg Jensen, M.; Matulevicius, V.; Zilaitiene, B.; Olesen, I.A.; Perheentupa, A.; Punab, M.; et al. Varicocele is associated with impaired semen quality and reproductive hormone levels: A study of 7035 healthy young men from six European countries. *Eur. Urol.* **2016**, *70*, 1019–1029. [CrossRef] [PubMed]
3. Akbay, E.; Cayan, S.; Doruk, E.; Duce, M.N.; Bozlu, M. The prevalence of varicocele and varicocele-related testicular atrophy in Turkish children and adolescents. *BJU Int.* **2000**, *86*, 490–493. [CrossRef] [PubMed]
4. Mongioì, L.M.; Mammino, L.; Compagnone, M.; Condorelli, R.A.; Basile, A.; Alamo, A.; La Vignera, S.; Morgia, G.; Russo, G.I.; Calogero, A.E. Effects of varicocele treatment on sperm conventional parameters: surgical varicocelectomy versus sclerotherapy. *Cardiovasc. Intervent. Radiol.* **2019**, *42*, 396–404. [CrossRef] [PubMed]
5. Kirby, E.W.; Wiener, L.E.; Rajanahally, S.; Crowell, K.; Coward, R.M. Undergoing varicocele repair before assisted reproduction improves pregnancy rate and live birth rate in azoospermic and oligospermic men with a varicocele: A systematic review and meta-analysis. *Fertil. Steril.* **2016**, *106*, 1338–1343. [CrossRef]
6. La Vignera, S.; Condorelli, R.; Vicari, E.; D'Agata, R.; Calogero, A.E. Effects of varicocelectomy on sperm DNA fragmentation, mitochondrial function, chromatin condensation, and apoptosis. *J. Androl.* **2012**, *33*, 389–396. [CrossRef]
7. Li, F.; Yue, H.; Yamaguchi, K.; Okada, K.; Matsushita, K.; Ando, M.; Chiba, K.; Fujisawa, M. Effect of surgical repair on testosterone production in infertile men with varicocele: A meta-analysis. *Int. J. Urol.* **2012**, *19*, 149–154. [CrossRef]
8. Cho, C.L.; Esteves, S.C.; Agarwal, A. Indications and outcomes of varicocele repair. *Panminerva Medica* **2019**, *61*, 152–163. [CrossRef]
9. Glassberg, K.I.; Korets, R. Update on the management of adolescent varicocele. *F1000 Med. Rep.* **2010**, *12*, 2. [CrossRef]

10. Chung, J.M.; Lee, S.D. Current issues in adolescent varicocele: Pediatric urological perspectives. *World J. Men's Health.* **2018**, *36*, 123–131. [CrossRef]
11. Nork, J.J.; Berger, J.H.; Crain, D.S.; Christman, M.S. Youth varicocele and varicocele treatment: A meta-analysis of semen outcomes. *Fertil. Steril.* **2014**, *102*, 381–387. [CrossRef] [PubMed]
12. Diamond, D.A.; Zurakowski, D.; Bauer, S.B.; Borer, J.G.; Peters, C.A.; Cilento, B.G., Jr.; Paltiel, H.J.; Rosoklija, I.; Retik, A.B. Relationship of varicocele grade and testicular hypotrophy to semen parameters in adolescents. *J. Urol.* **2007**, *178*, 1584–1588. [CrossRef] [PubMed]
13. Niu, X.B.; Tang, J.; Wang, H.B.; Yan, L.; Zhang, C.Y.; Wang, G.C.; Liang, J.; Dou, X.Y.; Fu, G.B. Inhibin B level helps evaluate the testicular function of prepubertal patients with varicocele. *Zhonghua Nan KeXue* **2018**, *24*, 618–621.
14. Gökçe, A.; Davarci, M.; Yalçinkaya, F.R.; Güven, E.O.; Kaya, Y.S.; Helvaci, M.R.; Balbay, M.D. Hereditary behavior of varicocele. *J. Androl.* **2010**, *31*, 288–290. [CrossRef] [PubMed]
15. Hassanin, A.M.; Ahmed, H.H.; Kaddah, A.N. A global view of the pathophysiology of varicocele. *Andrology* **2018**, *6*, 654–661. [CrossRef] [PubMed]
16. Condorelli, R.A.; Cannarella, R.; Calogero, A.E.; La Vignera, S. Evaluation of testicular function in prepubertal children. *Endocrine* **2018**, *62*, 274–280. [CrossRef] [PubMed]
17. Hu, J.T.; Shao, C.H.; Wang, P.T.; Liu, Y.; Hao, W.Y.; Feng, Y.L.; Liu, S.H.; Wang, X.S. High temperature reduces the proliferation of and occludin expression in rat Sertoli cells in vitro. *Zhonghua Nan KeXue* **2012**, *18*, 920–924.
18. Abdel-Meguid, T.A.; Al-Sayyad, A.; Tayib, A.; Farsi, H.M. Does varicocele repair improve male infertility? An evidence-based perspective from a randomized, controlled trial. *Eur. Urol.* **2011**, *59*, 455–461. [CrossRef]
19. Macey, M.R.; Owen, R.C.; Ross, S.S.; Coward, R.M. Best practice in the diagnosis and treatment of varicocele in children and adolescents. *Ther. Adv. Urol.* **2018**, *10*, 273–282. [CrossRef]
20. Dubin, L.; Amelar, R.D. Varicocele size and results of varicocelectomy in selected subfertile men with varicocele. *Fertil. Steril.* **1970**, *21*, 606–609. [CrossRef]
21. Condorelli, R.A.; Calogero, A.E.; Vicari, E.; Mongioi', L.; Burgio, G.; Cannarella, R.; Giacone, F.; Iacoviello, L.; Morgia, G.; Favilla, V.; et al. Reduced seminal concentration of CD45pos cells after follicle-stimulating hormone treatment in selected patients with idiopathic oligoasthenoteratozoospermia. *Int. J. Endocrinol.* **2014**, *2014*, 372060. [CrossRef] [PubMed]
22. Pauroso, S.; Di Leo, N.; Fulle, I.; Di Segni, M.; Alessi, S.; Maggini, E. Varicocele: Ultrasonographic assessment in dailyclinical practice. *J. Ultrasound.* **2011**, *14*, 199–204. [CrossRef] [PubMed]
23. Englund, K.M.; Rayment, M. Nutcracker syndrome: A proposed ultrasound protocol. *Australasian J. Ultrasound Med. Banner.* **2018**, *21*, 75–78. [CrossRef]
24. Hannick, J.H.; Blais, A.S.; Kim, J.K.; Traubici, J.; Shiff, M.; Book, R.; Lorenzo, A.J. Prevalence, doppler ultrasound findings, and clinical implications of the nutcracker phenomenon in pediatric varicoceles. *Urology* **2019**, *128*, 78–83. [CrossRef] [PubMed]
25. Jedrzejewski, G.; Osemlak, P.; Wieczorek, A.P.; Nachulewicz, P. Prognostic values of shear wave elastography in adolescent boys with varicocele. *J. Pediatr. Urol.* **2019**, *15*, e1–e5. [CrossRef]
26. Dabaja, A.A.; Wosnitzer, M.S.; Bolyakov, A.; Schlegel, P.N.; Paduch, D.A. When to ask male adolescents to provide semen sample for fertility preservation? *Transl. Androl. Urol.* **2014**, *3*, 2–8. [PubMed]
27. Fine, R.G.; Gitlin, J.; Reda, E.F.; Palmer, L.S. Barriers to use of semen analysis in the adolescent with a varicocele: Survey of patient, parental, and practitioner attitudes. *J. Pediatr. Urol.* **2016**, *12*, 41.e1–41.e6. [CrossRef]
28. Haans, L.C.; Laven, J.S.; Mali, W.P.; te Velde, E.R.; Wensing, C.J. Testis volumes, semen quality, and hormonal patterns in adolescents with and without a varicocele. *Fertil. Steril.* **1991**, *56*, 731–736. [CrossRef]
29. Paduch, D.A.; Niedzielski, J. Semen analysis in young men with varicocele: Preliminary study. *J. Urol.* **1996**, *156*, 788–790. [CrossRef]
30. Romeo, C.; Arrigo, T.; Impellizzeri, P.; Manganaro, A.; Antonuccio, P.; Di Pasquale, G.; Messina, M.F.; Marseglia, L.; Formica, I.; Zuccarello, B. Alteredseruminhibin b levels in adolescents with varicocele. *J. Pediatr. Surg.* **2007**, *42*, 390–394. [CrossRef]
31. Trigo, R.V.; Bergadá, I.; Rey, R.; Ballerini, M.G.; Bedecarrás, P.; Bergadá, C.; Gottlieb, S.; Campo, S. Altered serum profile of inhibin B, Pro-αC and anti-Müllerian hormone in prepubertal and pubertal boys with varicocele. *Clin. Endocrinol.* **2004**, *60*, 758–764. [CrossRef] [PubMed]

32. Chu, D.I.; Zderic, S.A.; Shukla, A.R.; Srinivasan, A.K.; Tasian, G.E.; Weiss, D.A.; Long, C.J.; Canning, D.A.; Kolon, T.F. The natural history of semen parameters in untreated asymptomatic adolescent varicocele patients: A retrospective cohort study. *J. Pediatr. Urol.* **2017**, *13*, 77.e1–77.e5. [CrossRef] [PubMed]
33. Kolon, T.F.; Clement, M.R.; Cartwright, L.; Bellah, R.; Carr, M.C.; Canning, D.A.; Snyder, H.M. Transient asynchronous testicular growth in adolescent males with a varicocele. *J. Urol.* **2008**, *180*, 1111–1114. [CrossRef] [PubMed]
34. Kozakowski, K.A.; Gjertson, C.K.; Decastro, G.J.; Poon, S.; Gasalberti, A.; Glassberg, K.I. Peak retrograde flow: A novel predictor of persistent, progressive and new onset asymmetry in adolescent varicocele. *J. Urol.* **2009**, *181*, 2717–2722. [CrossRef] [PubMed]
35. Van Batavia, J.P.; Badalato, G.; Fast, A.; Glassberg, K.I. Adolescent varicocele-is the 20/38 harbinger a durable predictor of testicular asymmetry? *J. Urol.* **2013**, *189*, 1897–1901. [CrossRef] [PubMed]
36. Cimador, M.; Castagnetti, M.; Gattuccio, I.; Pensabene, M.; Sergio, M.; De Grazia, E. The hemodynamic approach to evaluating adolescent varicocele. *Nat. Rev. Urol.* **2012**, *9*, 247–257. [CrossRef] [PubMed]
37. Glassberg, K.I. My indications for treatment of the adolescent varicocele (and why?). *Trans. Androl. Urol.* **2014**, *3*, 402–412.
38. Zhou, T.; Zhang, W.; Chen, Q.; Li, L.; Cao, H.; Xu, C.L.; Sun, Y.H. Effect of varicocelectomy on testis volume and semen parameters in adolescents: A meta-analysis. *Asian J. Androl.* **2015**, *17*, 1012–1016. [PubMed]
39. Locke, J.A.; Maryam, N.; Kourosh, A. Treatment of varicocele in children and adolescents: A systematic review and meta-analysis of randomized controlled trials. *J. Pediatr. Urol.* **2017**, *13*, 437–445. [CrossRef] [PubMed]
40. Silay, M.S.; Hoen, L.; Quadackaers, J.; Undre, S.; Bogaert, G.; Dogan, H.S.; Kocvara, R.; Nijman, R.J.M.; Radmayr, C.; Tekgul, S.; et al. Treatment of varicocele in children and adolescents: A systematic review and meta-analysis from the European association of urology/European Society for Paediatric Urology guidelines panel. *Eur. Urol.* **2019**, *75*, 448–461. [CrossRef] [PubMed]
41. Schwentner, C.; Radmayr, C.; Lunacek, A.; Gozzi, C.; Pinggera, G.M.; Neururer, R.; Oswald, J. Laparoscopic varicocele ligation in children and adolescents using isosulphan blue: A prospective randomized trial. *BJU Int.* **2006**, *98*, 861–865. [CrossRef] [PubMed]
42. Shiraishi, K.; Oka, S.; Matsuyama, H. Surgical comparison of subinguinal and high inguinal microsurgical varicocelectomy for adolescent varicocele. *Int. J. Urol.* **2016**, *23*, 338–342. [CrossRef] [PubMed]
43. Laven, J.S.; Haans, L.C.; Mali, W.P.; te Velde, E.R.; Wensing, C.J.; Eimers, J.M. Effects of varicocele treatment in adolescents: A randomized study. *Fertil. Steril.* **1992**, *58*, 756–762. [CrossRef]
44. Moursy, E.E.; El Dahshoury, M.Z.; Hussein, M.M.; Mourad, M.Z.; Badawy, A.A. Dilemma of adolescent varicocele: Long-term outcome in patients managed surgically and in patients managed expectantly. *J. Pediatr. Urol.* **2013**, *9*, 1018–1022. [CrossRef] [PubMed]
45. Paduch, D.A.; Niedzielski, J. Repair versus observation in adolescent varicocele: A prospective study. *J. Urol.* **1997**, *12*, 410–413. [CrossRef] [PubMed]
46. Yamamoto, M.; Hibi, H.; Katsuno, S.; Miyake, K. Effects of varicocelectomy on testis volume and semen parameters in adolescents: A randomized prospective study. *Nagoya J. Med. Sci.* **1995**, *58*, 127–132. [PubMed]
47. Çayan, S.; Şahin, S.; Akbay, E. Paternity rates and time to conception in adolescents with varicocele undergoing microsurgical varicocele repair vs observation only: A single institution experience with 408 patients. *J. Urol.* **2017**, *198*, 195–201. [CrossRef] [PubMed]
48. Bogaert, G.; Orye, C.; De Win, G. Pubertal screening and treatment for varicocele do not improve chance of paternity as adult. *J. Urol.* **2013**, *189*, 2298–2303. [CrossRef]
49. Dong, W.; Yao, Y.; Huang, H.; Han, J.; Zhao, X.; Huang, J. Surgical management of nutcracker phenomenon presenting as left varicocele in adolescents: A novel approach. *J. Pediatr. Urol.* **2014**, *10*, 424–429. [CrossRef]
50. Practice committee of the American society for reproductive medicine; Society for male reproduction and urology. Report on varicocele and infertility: A committee opinion. *Fertil. Steril.* **2014**, *102*, 1556–1560. [CrossRef]
51. Jungwirth, A.; Giwercman, A.; Tournaye, H.; Diemer, T.; Kopa, Z.; Dohle, G.; Krausz, C. European Association of Urology working group on male infertility. European Association of Urology guidelines on male infertility: The 2012 update. *Eur. Urol.* **2012**, *62*, 324–332. [CrossRef] [PubMed]

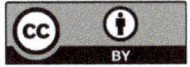

© 2019 by the authors. Licensee MDPI, Basel, Switzerland. This article is an open access article distributed under the terms and conditions of the Creative Commons Attribution (CC BY) license (http://creativecommons.org/licenses/by/4.0/).

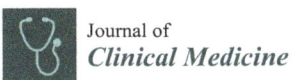 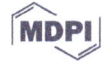

Journal of Clinical Medicine

Opinion

Early Identification of Isolated Sertoli Cell Dysfunction in Prepubertal and Transition Age: Is It Time?

Sandro La Vignera *, Rosita A. Condorelli, Laura Cimino, Rossella Cannarella, Filippo Giacone and Aldo E. Calogero

Department of Clinical and Experimental Medicine, University of Catania, 95123 Catania, Italy; rositacondorelli@unict.it (R.A.C.); lauracimino@hotmail.it (L.C.); roxcannarella@gmail.com (R.C.); filippogiacone@yahoo.it (F.G.); acaloger@unict.it (A.E.C.)
* Correspondence: sandrolavignera@unict.it

Received: 8 April 2019; Accepted: 7 May 2019; Published: 9 May 2019

Abstract: The male transitional phase is of fundamental importance for future fertility. This aspect is largely neglected in clinical practice. This opinion aims to shed light on these issues. The children frequently complete the transition phase with a slight reduction of testicular volume. The system of detecting testicular volume is often inadequate. These patients evidently complete puberty in an incomplete way because they do not reach an adequate testicular volume, albeit in the presence of adequate height and regular secondary sexual characteristics.

Keywords: primary prevention; male infertility; male transition

---

Male infertility is constantly growing [1], with an estimated prevalence of approximately 15% of couples of childbearing age in industrialized countries [2]. The male factor, alone or in combination with the female one, contributes in about half of the cases of couple infertility [1]. Worryingly, meta-regression analysis recently showed a substantial decrease of sperm concentration and total count in the last 40 years, whose causes have not yet been identified [3]. Therefore, further studies aimed at understanding the etiology of such decline as well as the adoption of prevention strategies are urgently needed.

The main interest has been mainly focused on secondary prevention strategies, mostly consisting in the treatment of the main diseases able to alter sperm quality (e.g., varicocele, urogenital infections, and endocrine disorders) [1,4,5]. Nevertheless, the evaluation of testicular function in prepubertal and transitional age would help in the early identification of testicular hypotrophy and signs of isolated tubulopathy and Sertoli cell (SC) dysfunction, thus timely recognizing a population at risk for male infertility. Accordingly, data from an epidemiological survey carried out in Italy by the Italian Society of Andrology and Medicine of Sexuality (SIAMS), revealed that 23% of 18 years old boys had low testicular volume (<12 mL) in a screening visit [6]. This evidence points to the importance of the adoption of measures aiming at evaluating testicular volume and function during the regular pediatric clinical practice. In this regard, the main concerns are when and how such investigation should be accomplished and which studies should be carried out to cover the limits of the current knowledge.

To allow a timely identification of isolated tubulopathy and SC dysfunction, the investigation should start in the prepubertal age and the transition phase. The latter is the moment of transition from the pediatrician to the family doctor [7]. It usually occurs around the age of 14 and is characterized by the following steps: (1) Increase of testicular volume (>4 mL at orchidometry); (2) Tanner II pubic hair; (3) growth spurt; (4) presence of spermatozoa in first morning urine; (5) Tanner V pubic hair [7]. Commonly, the lack of growth spurt and of secondary sexual characters appearance (both signs of insufficient testosterone production) are easily detectable, the failure to achieve an adequate testicular volume, a parameter closely associated with the fertility potential [8], is not frequently reported, apart from patients with significant testicular hypotrophy [7]. However, its detection is important for the primary prevention of male infertility (Figure 1).

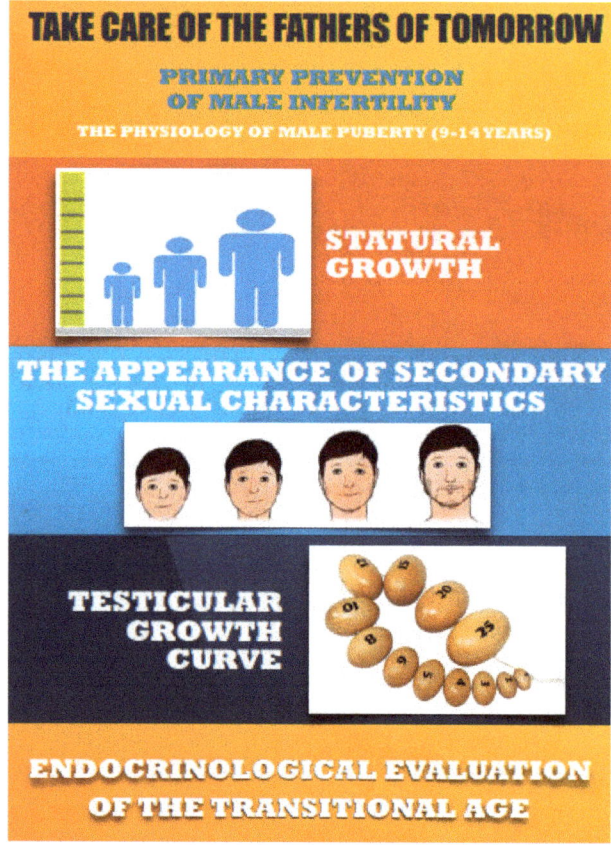

Figure 1. Primary prevention of male infertility. The importance of the testicular volume.

The normal testicular volume in adulthood ranges between 12 and 25 mL [8]. In the clinical practice, a slight testicular volume decrease (e.g., 8–12 mL) of unknown origin occurs more frequently than severe testicular hypotrophy. Testicular volume measurement is usually done by orchidometry which overestimates it compared to ultrasound evaluation. Despite the latter is much more accurate, it cannot be proposed to all patients [7,9,10]. Therefore, an electronic calculator has recently been developed from the Research Institute at Nationwide Children's Hospital to match ultrasound values. It requires the width of the testis, which may easily be obtained with a centimeter (cm) ruler at the physical examination, matched with the genital stage of development (G1 to G5) to elaborate a volume corresponding to each different phase of pubertal development [11]. Testicular volume nomogram and volume variations occurring in the transition through each stage of puberty in boys with normal and with delayed puberty have been described in a longitudinal study from a Danish cohort [12]. Testicular volumes expected according to the Tanner stage are reported in Table 1 [11].

Table 1. Testicular volume values according to the Tanner stage. Legend: The testicular volume is reported as median value [11].

Tanner Stage	Testicular Volume (mL)
I	0.71
II	3.62
III	6.42
IV	10.85
V	17.32

Beyond the testicular volume, the evaluation of SC function deserves further attention. The hypothalamic-pituitary-gonadal axis is almost quiescent by definition in the prepubertal phase [13]. This make gonadotropins not representative of testicular dysfunction at this age. By contrast, gonadotropins are commonly adopted in the clinical practice to diagnose hypogonadism in adulthood. Therefore, additional markers are needed.

The quiescence of the hypothalamic-pituitary-gonadal axis before puberty does not implicate a lack of endocrine testicular function. Indeed, the testis is mainly made of immature SCs in childhood. These are nurse cells displaying a pivotal role in spermatogenesis. Accordingly, they provide functional support to germ cells, their nourishment and defense, through both SC-based blood-testis-barrier and the secretion of immunomodulatory factors. Before puberty, immature SCs actively proliferate and secrete large amounts of antimüllerian hormone (AMH), whose extent reflect the maturation degree of SCs. When puberty starts, SCs move from a proliferative and immature phase to a quiescent and mature one and start to express the androgen receptor. Concomitantly, AMH levels decrease. SCs secrete also inhibin B, whose production depends on follicle-stimulating hormone (FSH)-stimulation. Therefore, inhibin B serum levels physiologically increase after puberty [7].

Both AMH and inhibin B could be adopted for the evaluation of SC function in prepubertal and transitional phase.

Low AMH levels in childhood reflect a SC dysfunction. Indeed, AMH levels depend on SC number and integrity. Low levels have been found in primary testicular disorders, such as cryptorchidism. In greater detail, low AMH levels have been found in 75% of children with bilateral cryptorchidism and nonpalpable testis and in 35% of those with inguinal testis [14]. Furthermore, the failure to have low AMH levels in the final stages of puberty expresses a condition of Sertolian functional immaturity, which possibly reflects decreased testosterone intratubular concentrations. The careful observation of the evolution of AMH levels in the course of pubertal development would allow us to receive the following information: (1) Adequate biological action of FSH; (2) adequate Sertolian proliferation; (3) appropriate expression of the androgen receptor by the SCs (functional maturity index); (4) adequate intratesticular biological action of testosterone [7]. These considerations highlight the importance of AMH measurement in prepubertal and transitional phase to timely identify any sign of SC dysfunction, responsible for primary testicular tubulopathy.

Noteworthy are also the results coming from a study carried out on male patients with central hypogonadism, where FSH stimulation resulted in an increase of AMH levels [15]. These findings suggest that an increase of AMH levels after FSH administration occurs in the presence of normal SC function (which is typical in central hypogonadism). Therefore, a stimulation test (after standardization and identification of cut-off levels) might be proposed in childhood when SC dysfunction is suspected.

The limits of AMH measurements should, however, be taken into account. Currently, it is performed by chemoluminescence. The specificity and sensitivity of the determination must be improved due to the absence of international reference standard, lack of comparability with the results of previous kit, and doubts about stability during the sample storage. Nonetheless, there are several evidences that allow us to know the normal values and the expected variations during puberty [16].

The significance of inhibin B levels have been also investigated in prepubertal and transition phase [17,18]. Low levels mainly reflect a defective FSH secretion and are useful in the differential diagnosis between congenital central hypogonadism and pubertal delay [19,20]. As far as its role in the early detection of a primary tubular dysfunction, low levels have been described in children with monolateral cryptorchidism compared to healthy ones [21,22], as well as in those with vanishing testis [22]. Therefore, they might represent a marker of SC integrity.

The possible role of insulin-like growth factor 1 (IGF1) for the achievement of testicular volume and function has been reported in experimental animals [23], but it requires further investigation in human being, especially in the light of the observed IGF1-induced SC proliferation in prepubertal animals [24].

Definitely, there is still the need to improve the reliability of testicular function parameters in prepubertal times, able to anticipate the diagnosis of testicular suffering, in particular the inadequate Sertolian function.

Further limits of the current practice deserving investigation regard the individuation of children at risk for the development of primary testicular tubulopathy. These include cryptorchidism, occurring in 2–4% of full-term and in 20–30% of premature births [25,26]; micropenis (which may hide partial androgen insensitivity syndrome even when present in isolated form) [27] and protracted hypoglycemia (pituitary disorders) [28]. Another less discussed topic concerns the possible cases of deficiency of minipuberty (physiological window of transient activation of the testicular pituitary gland in the neonatal period) characterized by increased levels of gonadotropins and testosterone [29]. The determination of INSL-3 (testicular hormone involved in the descent of the testicle in the fetal age) in children with cryptorchidism would allow us to have a marker that anticipates the decline of testosterone levels [30]. In addition, the offspring of mothers with gestational diabetes may be at risk for testicular tubulopathy predisposing to the development of cryptorchidism. Accordingly, a recent meta-analysis confirms an increased risk of cryptorchidism in births of mothers with gestational diabetes. The possible mechanism may be related to the decreased serum concentrations of sex hormone-binding globulin (SHBG) which cause the increase of free 17ß-estradiol and, in turn, undercut the production of INSL-3 [31].

More than 42 million overweight children were reported in 2014, with the prevalence doubling from 1980 to 2014 [32]. Whether obesity or hyperinsulinemia, both being widespread conditions in the pediatric population, especially in low- and middle-income countries [33], may affect SC function deserve to be investigated.

Prepubertal male obesity in Tanner stage II already causes a decreased Leydig cell function [34]. Insulin has direct effects on spermatozoa where it finds adequate presence of glucose transporters and where it favors the availability of lactate within the SC for the production of energy. In particular, the expression of MCT4 (lactate transporter from the SC to the intratubular space for subsequent internalization within the germ cells) is under the control of insulin [35]. Insulin resistance is increased in patients with unexplained infertility [36,37]. Interestingly, inhibin B levels have been found to decline with increasing obesity in young men [38]. Furthermore, AMH and inhibin B levels have been found lower in obese adolescents with insulin resistance compared to normal weight controls. Therefore, obesity and insulin resistance may impact on SC function in prepubertal boys [39].

In summary, the evaluation of testicular volume and of markers of SC function in prepubertal and transitional age are of importance for the precocious identification of signs of primary testicular tubulopathy. A flowchart that may be used in the clinical practice is showed in Figure 2. Children at risk for testicular tubulopathy, including those with testicular hypotrophy, should undergo to AMH and inhibin B serum measurement. In case of normal values, the testicular volume should be measured at least every six months and should be framed in the context of the other auxological parameters till a sperm analysis can be requested (1.5 years after the onset of puberty [40]). In case of abnormal AMH or inhibin B values, a stimulation test with FSH might be proposed in the future after proper standardization [15]. The lack of response might represent indication for treatment with FSH since the vast majority of cases with testicular tubulopathy have FSH serum levels within the normal range [41].

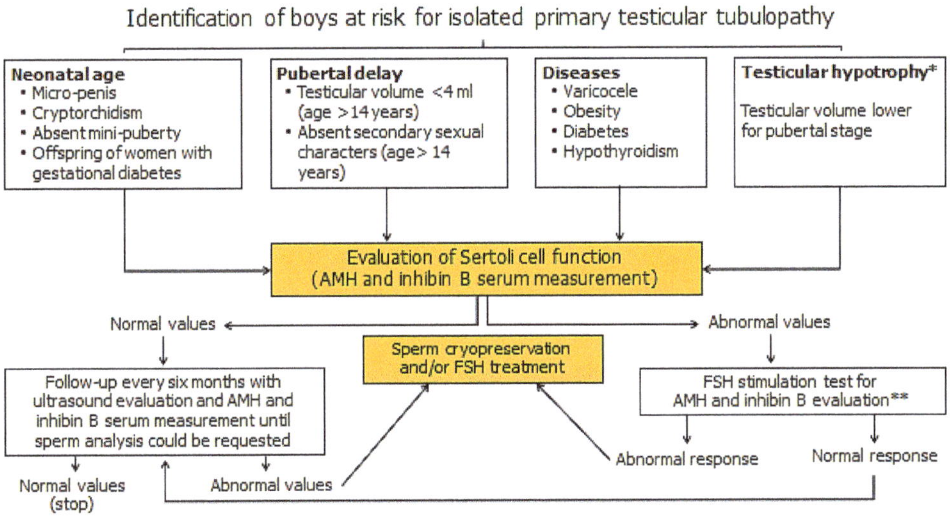

Figure 2. Flowchart proposed to help identify early testicular primary testicular tubulopathy in prepubertal and transitional age. * [42]; ** [15].

Conflicts of Interest: The authors declare no conflict of interest.

References

1. Duca, Y.; Calogero, A.E.; Cannarella, R.; Condorelli, R.A.; La Vignera, S. Current and emerging medical therapeutic agents for idiopathic male infertility. *Expert Opin. Pharmacother.* **2019**, *20*, 55–67. [CrossRef] [PubMed]
2. Agarwal, A.; Mulgund, A.; Hamada, A.; Chyatte, M.R. A unique view on male infertility around the globe. *Reprod. Biol. Endocrinol.* **2015**, *13*, 37. [CrossRef]
3. Levine, H.; Jørgensen, N.; Martino-Andrade, A.; Mendiola, J.; Weksler-Derri, D.; Mindlis, I.; Pinotti, R.; Swan, S.H. Temporal trends in sperm count: A systematic review and meta-regression analysis. *Hum. Reprod. Update* **2017**, *23*, 646–659. [CrossRef] [PubMed]
4. La Vignera, S.; Condorelli, R.; Vicari, E.; D'Agata, R.; Calogero, A.E. Effects of varicocelectomy on sperm DNA fragmentation, mitochondrial function, chromatin condensation, and apoptosis. *J. Androl.* **2012**, *33*, 389–396. [CrossRef]
5. Condorelli, R.A.; Russo, G.I.; Calogero, A.E.; Morgia, G.; La Vignera, S. Chronic prostatitis and its detrimental impact on sperm parameters: A systematic review and meta-analysis. *J. Endocrinol. Investig.* **2017**, *40*, 1209–1218. [CrossRef]
6. Foresta, C.; Garolla, A.; Frigo, A.C.; Carraro, U.; Isidori, A.M.; Lenzi, A.; Ferlin, A. Anthropometric, penile and testis measures in post-pubertal Italian males. *J. Endocrinol. Investig.* **2013**, *36*, 287–292.
7. Condorelli, R.A.; Cannarella, R.; Calogero, A.E.; La Vignera, S. Evaluation of testicular function in prepubertal children. *Endocrine* **2018**, *62*, 274–280. [CrossRef]
8. Condorelli, R.; Calogero, A.E.; La Vignera, S. Relationship between Testicular Volume and Conventional or Nonconventional Sperm Parameters. *Int. J. Endocrinol.* **2013**, *2013*, 145792. [CrossRef]
9. Sakamoto, H.; Ogawa, Y.; Yoshida, H. Relationship between testicular volume and testicular function: Comparison of the Prader orchidometric and ultrasonographic measurements in patients with infertility. *Asian J. Androl.* **2008**, *10*, 319–324. [CrossRef]
10. Goede, J.; Hack, W.W.; Sijstermans, K.; Van der Voort-Doedens, L.M.; Van der Ploeg, T.; Meij-de Vries, A.; Delemarre-van de Waal, H.A. Normative values for testicular volume measured by ultrasonography in a normal population from infancy to adolescence. *Horm. Res. Paediatr.* **2011**, *76*, 56–64. [CrossRef]

11. Sotos, J.F.; Tokar, N.J. A medical calculator to determine testicular volumes matching ultrasound values from the width of the testis obtained in the scrotum with a centimeter ruler. *Int. J. Pediatr. Endocrinol.* **2017**, *2017*, 14. [CrossRef]
12. Lawaetz, J.G.; Hagen, C.P.; Mieritz, M.G.; Blomberg Jensen, M.; Petersen, J.H.; Juul, A. Evaluation of 451 Danish boys with delayed puberty: Diagnostic use of a new puberty nomogram and effects of oral testosterone therapy. *J. Clin. Endocrinol. Metab.* **2015**, *100*, 1376–1385. [CrossRef] [PubMed]
13. Grinspon, R.P.; Urrutia, M.; Rey, R.A. Male Central Hypogonadism in Paediatrics—The Relevance of Follicle-stimulating Hormone and Sertoli Cell Markers. *Eur. Endocrinol.* **2018**, *14*, 67–71. [CrossRef]
14. Misra, M.; MacLaughlin, D.T.; Donahoe, P.K.; Lee, M.M. Measurement of Mullerian inhibiting substance facilitates management of boys with microphallus and cryptorchidism. *J. Clin. Endocrinol. Metab.* **2002**, *87*, 3598–3602. [CrossRef] [PubMed]
15. Young, J.; Chanson, P.; Salenave, S.; Noël, M.; Brailly, S.; O'Flaherty, M.; Schaison, G.; Rey, R. Testicular anti-mullerian hormone secretion is stimulated by recombinant human FSH in patients with congenital hypogonadotropic hypogonadism. *J. Clin. Endocrinol. Metab.* **2005**, *90*, 724–728. [CrossRef] [PubMed]
16. Edelsztein, N.Y.; Grinspon, R.P.; Schteingart, H.F.; Rey, R.A. Anti-Müllerian hormone as a marker of steroid and gonadotropin action in the testis of children and adolescents with disorders of the gonadal axis. *Int. J. Pediatr. Endocrinol.* **2016**, *2016*, 20. [CrossRef] [PubMed]
17. Johansen, M.L.; Anand-Ivell, R.; Mouritsen, A.; Hagen, C.P.; Mieritz, M.G.; Søeborg, T.; Johannsen, T.H.; Main, K.M.; Andersson, A.M.; Ivell, R.; et al. Serum levels of insulin-like factor 3, anti-Mullerian hormone, inhibin B, and testosterone during pubertal transition in healthy boys: A longitudinal pilot study. *Reproduction* **2014**, *147*, 529–535. [CrossRef]
18. Grinspon, R.P.; Loreti, N.; Braslavsky, D.; Valeri, C.; Schteingart, H.; Ballerini, M.G.; Bedecarrás, P.; Ambao, V.; Gottlieb, S.; Ropelato, M.G.; et al. Spreading the clinical window for diagnosing fetal-onset hypogonadism in boys. *Front. Endocrinol.* **2014**, *5*, 51. [CrossRef]
19. Binder, G.; Schweizer, R.; Blumenstock, G.; Braun, R. Inhibin B plus LH vs GnRH agonist test for distinguishing constitutional delay of growth and puberty from isolated hypogonadotropic hypogonadism in boys. *Clin. Endocrinol.* **2015**, *82*, 100–105. [CrossRef]
20. Rohayem, J.; Nieschlag, E.; Kliesch, S.; Zitzmann, M. Inhibin B, AMH, but not INSL3, IGF1 or DHEAS support differentiation between constitutional delay of growth and puberty and hypogonadotropic hypogonadism. *Andrology* **2015**, *3*, 882–887. [CrossRef]
21. Cao, S.S.; Shan, X.O.; Hu, Y.Y. Impact of unilateral cryptorchidism on the levels of serum anti-müllerian hormone and inhibin B. *Zhonghua Nan KeXue* **2016**, *22*, 805–808.
22. Thorup, J.; Kvist, K.; Clasen-Linde, E.; Hutson, J.M.; Cortes, D. Serum inhibin B values in boys with unilateral vanished testis or unilateral cryptorchidism. *J. Urol.* **2015**, *193*, 1632–1636. [CrossRef]
23. Cannarella, R.; Condorelli, R.A.; La Vignera, S.; Calogero, A.E. Effects of the insulin-like growth factor system on testicular differentiation and function: A review of the literature. *Andrology* **2018**, *6*, 3–9. [CrossRef]
24. Dance, A.; Kastelic, J.; Thundathil, J. A combination of insulin-like growth factor I (IGF-I) and FSH promotes proliferation of prepubertal bovine Sertoli cells isolated and cultured in vitro. *Reprod. Fertil. Dev.* **2017**, *29*, 1635–1641. [CrossRef] [PubMed]
25. La Vignera, S.; Calogero, A.E.; Condorelli, R.; Marziani, A.; Cannizzaro, M.A.; Lanzafame, F.; Vicari, E. Cryptorchidism and its long-term complications. *Eur. Rev. Med. Pharmacol. Sci.* **2009**, *13*, 351–356.
26. Ferlin, A.; Zuccarello, D.; Zuccarello, B.; Chirico, M.R.; Zanon, G.F.; Foresta, C. Genetic alterations associated with cryptorchidism. *JAMA* **2008**, *300*, 2271–2276. [CrossRef]
27. Bhangoo, A.; Paris, F.; Philibert, P.; Audran, F.; Ten, S.; Sultan, C. Isolated micropenis reveals partial androgen insensitivity syndrome confirmed by molecular analysis. *Asian J. Androl.* **2010**, *12*, 561–566. [CrossRef] [PubMed]
28. Yong, S.C.; Boo, N.Y.; Wu, L.L. Persistent neonatal hypoglycaemia as a result of hypoplastic pituitary gland. *Br. J. Hosp. Med.* **2006**, *67*, 326. [CrossRef]
29. Swee, D.S.; Quinton, R. Congenital Hypogonadotrophic Hypogonadism: Minipuberty and the Case for Neonatal Diagnosis. *Front. Endocrinol.* **2019**, *10*, 97. [CrossRef]
30. Ferlin, A.; Simonato, M.; Bartoloni, L.; Rizzo, G.; Bettella, A.; Dottorini, T.; Dallapiccola, B.; Foresta, C. The INSL3-LGR8/GREAT ligand-receptor pair in human cryptorchidism. *J. Clin. Endocrinol. Metab.* **2003**, *88*, 4273–4279. [CrossRef] [PubMed]

31. Zhang, L.; Wang, X.H.; Zheng, X.M.; Liu, T.Z.; Zhang, W.B.; Zheng, H.; Chen, M.F. Maternal gestational smoking, diabetes, alcohol drinking, pre-pregnancy obesity and the risk of cryptorchidism: A systematic review and meta-analysis of observational studies. *PLoS ONE* **2015**, *10*, e0119006. [CrossRef]
32. WHO Obesity and Overweight 2016. Available online: http://www.who.int/mediacentre/factsheets/fs311/en/ (accessed on 15 April 2019).
33. Farpour-Lambert, N.J.; Baker, J.L.; Hassapidou, M.; Holm, J.C.; Nowicka, P.; O'Malley, G.; Weiss, R. Childhood obesity is a chronic disease demanding specific health care-a position statement from the Childhood Obesity Task Force (COTF) of the European Association for the Study of Obesity (EASO). *Obes. Facts* **2015**, *8*, 342–349. [CrossRef]
34. Condorelli, R.A.; Calogero, A.E.; Vicari, E.; Mongioi', L.; Favilla, V.; Morgia, G.; Cimino, S.; Russo, G.; La Vignera, S. The gonadal function in obese adolescents: Review. *J. Endocrinol. Investig.* **2014**, *37*, 1133–1142. [CrossRef] [PubMed]
35. Alves, M.G.; Martins, A.D.; Rato, L.; Moreira, P.I.; Socorro, S.; Oliveira, P.F. Molecular mechanisms beyond glucose transport in diabetes-related male infertility. *Biochim. Biophys. Acta* **2013**, *1832*, 626–635. [CrossRef]
36. Mansour, R.; El-Faissal, Y.; Kamel, A.; Kamal, O.; Aboulserour, G.; Aboulghar, M.; Fahmy, I. Increased insulin resistance in men with unexplained infertility. *Reprod. Biomed. Online* **2017**, *35*, 571–575. [CrossRef] [PubMed]
37. Campbell, J.M.; Lane, M.; Owens, J.A.; Bakos, H.W. Paternal obesity negatively affects male fertility and assisted reproduction outcomes: A systematic review and meta-analysis. *Reprod. Biomed. Online* **2015**, *31*, 593–604. [CrossRef]
38. Winters, S.J.; Wang, C.; Abdelrahaman, E.; Hadeed, V.; Dyky, M.A.; Brufsky, A. Inhibin-B levels in healthy young adult men and prepubertal boys: Is obesity the cause for the contemporary decline in sperm count because of fewer Sertoli cells? *J. Androl.* **2006**, *27*, 560–564. [CrossRef] [PubMed]
39. Buyukinan, M.; Atar, M.; Pirgon, O.; Kurku, H.; Erdem, S.S.; Deniz, I. Anti-Mullerian Hormone and Inhibin B Levels in Obese Boys; Relations with Cardiovascular Risk Factors. *Exp. Clin. Endocrinol. Diabetes* **2018**, *126*, 528–533. [CrossRef]
40. Dabaja, A.A.; Wosnitzer, M.S.; Bolyakov, A.; Schlegel, P.N.; Paduch, D.A. When to ask male adolescents to provide semen sample for fertility preservation? *Transl. Androl. Urol.* **2014**, *3*, 2–8.
41. La Vignera, S.; Condorelli, R.A.; Duca, Y.; Mongioi, L.M.; Cannarella, R.; Giacone, F.; Calogero, A.E. FSH therapy for idiopathic male infertility: Four schemes are better than one. *Aging Male* **2019**, *3*, 1–6. [CrossRef]
42. Testicular Volume Calculator. Available online: http://tvcalculator.nchri.org (accessed on 15 April 2019).

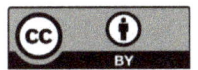

© 2019 by the authors. Licensee MDPI, Basel, Switzerland. This article is an open access article distributed under the terms and conditions of the Creative Commons Attribution (CC BY) license (http://creativecommons.org/licenses/by/4.0/).

MDPI
St. Alban-Anlage 66
4052 Basel
Switzerland
Tel. +41 61 683 77 34
Fax +41 61 302 89 18
www.mdpi.com

Journal of Clinical Medicine Editorial Office
E-mail: jcm@mdpi.com
www.mdpi.com/journal/jcm

www.ingramcontent.com/pod-product-compliance
Lightning Source LLC
LaVergne TN
LVHW070555100526
838202LV00012B/475